EARLY EVENTS IN DIABETIC RETINOPATHY AND INTERVENTION STRATEGIES

Edited by **Andrew T.C. Tsin**
and **Jeffery G. Grigsby**

Early Events in Diabetic Retinopathy and Intervention Strategies
http://dx.doi.org/10.5772/intechopen.69906
Edited by Andrew T.C. Tsin and Jeffery G. Grigsby

Contributors

Julia Hafner, Ursula Schmidt-Erfurth, Sonja Karst, Ashwath Jayagopal, Derrick Feenstra, Faye Drawnel, Kevin Bermea, Andrew Tsin, Andi Arus Victor, Ratna Sitompul

Notice

First published in London, United Kingdom, 2018 by IntechOpen
IntechOpen is the global imprint of INTECHOPEN LIMITED, registered in England and Wales, registration number: 11086078, The Shard, 25th floor, 32 London Bridge Street
London, SE19SG – United Kingdom
Printed in Croatia

British Library Cataloguing-in-Publication Data
A catalogue record for this book is available from the British Library

Additional hard copies can be obtained from orders@intechopen.com

Early Events in Diabetic Retinopathy and Intervention Strategies, Edited by Andrew T.C. Tsin and Jeffery G. Grigsby
p. cm.
Print ISBN 978-1-78923-082-6
Online ISBN 978-1-78923-083-3

For EU product safety concerns:
IN TECH d.o.o., Prolaz Marije Krucifikse Kozulić 3, 51000 Rijeka, Croatia,
info@intechopen.com or visit our website at intechopen.com.

Meet the editors

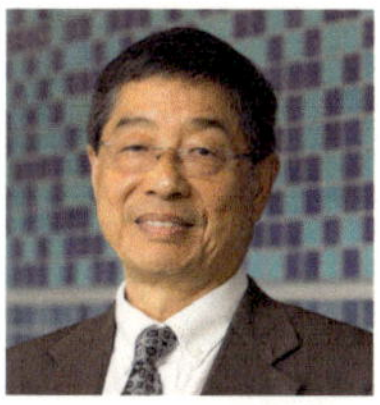

Professor Andrew Tsin is the Chair of Biomedical Sciences Department and the Associate Dean of Research, School of Medicine, at the University of Texas Rio Grande Valley in Edinburg, Texas. His laboratory conducts research to study visual pigment regeneration and ocular diseases from diabetic complications. Professor Tsin has published more than 300 refereed research articles and conference papers. He is a Gold Fellow of the Association for Research in Vision and Ophthalmology, a Fellow of the Royal Society of Medicine, and a Fellow of the American Association for the Advancement of Science. In 2011, Professor Tsin was presented a Presidential Award for Excellence in Science, Mathematics and Engineering Mentoring by President Obama at the Oval Office.

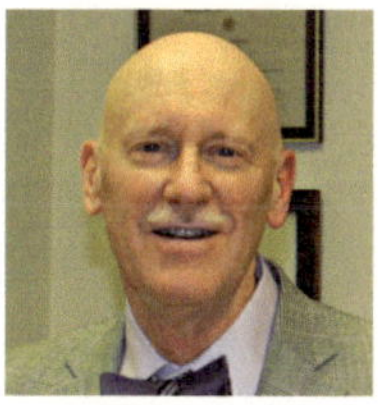

Jeffery G. Grigsby is a practicing optometrist, biologist, researcher, and writer with a special interest in diabetic eye disease. In his earlier career, he provided patient care in optometric and ophthalmologic practices in West Texas. He chaired or served on 18 different Texas Optometric Association (TOA) committees and served as the president of that organization. He is a four-time recipient of the TOA's Presidential Award for Service. In a mid-career shift, he currently divides his time between seeing patients, doing research, writing reviews on special interest topics in diabetic eye disease, and teaching. Currently, he serves as an adjunct faculty member at the University of Houston, College of Optometry, and a recurrent faculty member at the Texas Tech University Health Sciences Center.

Contents

Preface

The causative agents of type 1 and type 2 diabetes differ, but the main dysfunction by which they inflict damage to the human body is the same: hyperglycemia. Other systemic factors such as hypertension, lipid levels, and genetics also contribute to the effects diabetes has on individuals afflicted with this condition. Our ability in health care to control these factors has improved, but still those with diabetes too often suffer from kidney disease, neuropathy, amputation, and diabetic retinopathy. It is expected that in 20 years' duration nearly all those with diabetes will exhibit some diabetic retinopathy. In some patients, it will progress to blindness.

Currently, the only treatment available in the early stages of diagnosis and treatment of diabetes to control diabetic retinopathy is management of the above-listed systemic factors. Diabetic retinopathy is a slow process beginning with early damage to retinal vasculature and retinal ganglion cells. Often, years of damage to the diabetic retina occurs before it progresses to a level where our current treatments of diabetic retinopathy play a role. Pan-retinal photocoagulation has stood the test of time helping reduce the risk of blindness, but it leaves the patient with reduced vision, especially at night. Injections of anti-VEGF agents have shown to be effective in many cases of diabetic macular edema. In addition, they have demonstrated effectiveness in treating proliferative diabetic retinopathy; however, many questions remain regarding the wisdom of using anti-VEGF agents for extended periods of time on these relatively young individuals.

The number of those diagnosed with type 2 diabetes in both developed and developing countries has sky-rocketed. It is expected that the prevalence of individuals with type 2 diabetes will continue to increase. Healthcare systems in these countries struggle to screen those at risk of diabetic retinopathy who have either type 1 or type 2 diabetes.

This book covers topics addressing imaging processes currently available in the development stage for screening of diabetic retinopathy. It also covers potential biomarkers that may be used to identify those at risk. Further, new pathways which can lead to diabetic retinopathy are identified.

We are grateful to those contributors who have labored to make this book a reality. We would also like to thank the staff at InTech, especially Marina Dusevic, Publishing Process Manager, who helped us through this process. It is our hope that this book will serve as a resource for clinicians, scientists, and public health workers by expanding knowledge on diabetic retinopathy, as well as offering insights into the screening modalities, which might help those developing the condition. Further, it is also our hope that this book will offer illumination into the early mechanisms of diabetes and help us identify targets that, if addressed early enough, might prevent us from ever having to use our present treatment procedures.

Jeffery G. Grigsby
Vision Health Specialties, Midland, Texas, USA
College of Optometry, University of Houston, Houston, Texas, USA
Texas Tech University Health Science Center, Midland, Texas, USA

Andrew T.C. Tsin
Department of Biomedical Sciences
University of Texas Rio Grande Valley, School of Medicine
Edinberg, Texas, USA

Section 1

Introduction

Chapter 1

Introductory Chapter: Diabetes, It is Always Something

Jeffery G. Grigsby and Andrew T.C. Tsin

Additional information is available at the end of the chapter

http://dx.doi.org/10.5772/intechopen.75687

1. Where we are and how we got there

The diabetes world changed when Banting and Best reported on their success extracting insulin from a dog in 1922. Previous to that, the diagnosis of type 1 diabetes was a death sentence. In the 1800s, a 10-year-old diagnosed with type 1 diabetes would wither away and die within a year. When the two Canadians extracted insulin, a very dark cloud lifted.

6:00 AM, the alarm goes off. Time to get up and start another day. Shower, dress, and check blood glucose for the first time that day. A little low this morning. I will have to eat a little extra or cut back on the insulin some. Cereal, milk, and juice for breakfast. A bowl of cereal, 32 g of carbohydrate, 20 g of milk, and 30 g of juice. 82 g in total; ratios vary between patients, but let us use 1 unit of fast acting insulin for every 10 g of carbohydrate, so normally that would be 8.2 units of insulin to cover breakfast. Since we are starting a little low, let us just inject 6 units to cover the meal and the low. On and on all day. Every day. No time off just because it is Thanksgiving or your first date.

Diabetes is still no piece of cake. It is difficult, but doable. Today we even have a U.S. Supreme Court Justice with nearly life-long (diagnosis age 7) type 1 diabetes. Maintaining normal levels of blood glucose are a constant challenge to those with type 1 diabetes. In fact, achieving blood glucose levels equivalent to those considered normal for those without diabetes, may not even be a desirable goal. There are too many lows and then there is the Action to Control Cardiovascular Risk in Diabetes Study (ACCORD) which told us those levels may not even advisable.

Type 2 diabetes is at epidemic levels in both developed and developing countries. Still the battle to level the highs and lows is difficult, but manageable; however, many do not even know they have it and many do not have the resources or knowledge to deal with it.

With longer lives we found there could be complications such as eye, kidney, and extremity issues that did not show up when a diabetes life span was less than a year. The problems are present in those cells not requiring insulin as the gate keeper into the cell. Nearly every scientific paper written on diabetic retinopathy has an introduction telling the reader that diabetes is the leading cause of blindness in the working age population. Most of them maintain their vision, but some do not, even in countries with excellent health care systems.

2. Mechanisms, research, screening, and the future

Research into diabetes is also complicated by the lack of a good animal model. There are many animals which can simulate human diabetes, but none demonstrate the full blown aberrant retinal blood vessel development that can occur in someone with diabetes of many years duration. Perhaps the animal models do not live long enough to exhibit this type of damage.

Refractive changes may be one of the presenting signs of increased blood glucose; usually a move toward more myopia or less hyperopia. Cataract is also more likely to develop and does so earlier in poorly controlled diabetes. Diabetic retinopathy takes years to develop, although poorly controlled systemic factors and pregnancy can speed up the process. Blood glucose levels, especially A1c, blood pressure, lipid levels, and genetics all play a role in determining who will or will not develop retinopathy complications.

Diabetic retinopathy is a gradual process whose mechanism of action is not totally understood. It seems to start with damage to retinal ganglion cells and retinal capillaries. Hyperglycemia can result in the production of reactive oxygen species, hyperosmolarity of cells, production of advanced glycation products, activation of protein kinase C, retinal inflammation, and increased production of nitric oxide, which may individually or collectively play a role in the development of diabetic retinopathy. Retinal capillaries are lined with endothelial cells and pericytes which depend on each other for support. One of the initial steps occurring with hyperglycemia in the retina is the damage and loss of pericytes. Without the support supplied by pericytes, endothelial cells will eventually die leaving acellular capillaries or those damaged to the point where they no longer bring oxygen and remove carbon dioxide from retinal cells. It should be pointed out that the oxygen demand of retinal cells greatly exceeds than that of other cells in the body. As a response, cells starved for oxygen accumulate hypoxia inducible factor (HIF) which stimulates the production of vascular endothelial growth factor (VEGF) that initiates the formation of new blood vessels. One would think this might be a positive factor, except these poorly developed vessels leak, hemorrhage, and grow into the vitreous. When the vitreous shifts, this can pull the neural retina loose from its attachment to the retinal pigment epithelium (RPE) resulting in (a very difficult to fix) retinal detachment. At times, this can result in blindness.

Clinically, diabetic retinopathy is broken down into non-proliferative (NPDR) and proliferative retinopathy (PDR); proliferative indicating the development of new blood vessels. It is a continuum, from the initial hyperglycemia to damaged leaky vessels to the production of new blood vessels in response to hypoxia. The early damage of these vessels is visible viewing the ocular fundus as the small dots of hemorrhages and microaneursyms. Later on the vessel damage progresses to a point where blood, fats, and other fluids from the retina leak into the retina. One possible complication of this is diabetic macular edema (DME). The fluid accumulating in the retina can damage an individual's central vision. For many years, macular laser has been the preferred treatment for DME, but newer trials have exhibited the effectiveness of anti-VEGF agents in helping control this complication. Sometimes anti-VEGFs are ineffective indicating that factors other than VEGF may play a role in the development of DME. DME can be a complication of both NPDR and PDR and can result in temporary, and in some cases, permanent vision impairment.

For many years, the primary procedure used to prevent blindness once PDR begins has been pan-retinal photocoagulation (PRP), which is a series of laser burns scattered over the retina. It is effective because it reduces oxygen demand of the retina by eliminating retinal neuronal elements and increases oxygen perfusion from the outer lying choroid. Unfortunately it reduces best corrected central vision as well as peripheral and night vision. Currently, the use of anti-VEGF injections is being investigated in an attempt to reduce or eliminate PDR, either in addition to, or in place of PRP, but many questions remain as to its long-term effects. Is this only a short-term treatment? Does the underlying causative hypoxia persist after treatment? Some studies have shown destruction of retinal components with long-term use of anti-VEGF injections. Are we causing degeneration of the retina in this relatively younger population of patients?

The Diabetes Control and Complications Trial (DCCT) told us that the higher the percentage of glycated hemoglobin, or A1c, the higher the risk of developing DR. This increase of DR with increasing A1c occurs not linearly, but in an exponential fashion. The United Kingdom Prospective Diabetes Study, done primarily on type 2 diabetes patients, found a positive effect of intensive blood pressure (BP) control. Further evaluation in the ACCORD study found no additional benefit of lowering BP below the long-standing limit of 140/90. However, more recently, the American College of Cardiology and the American Heart Association, in an effort to reduce the risk of heart attack and stroke, have reset the blood pressure desirable normal below this to 130/80. In addition, ACCORD demonstrated a decrease in the need for focal laser for DME with the use of fenofibrate to reduce triglycerides. Fenofibrate has been approved by Australian authorities to treat DR.

As previously mentioned, rates of type 2 diabetes have soared in both developed and developing countries outnumbering the number of professionals available to screen for DR. Many screening programs have been tried or are under investigation, but so far they have been inadequate in real world situations. Thus, the attempt to implement better screening modalities in underserved urban and rural areas is a much desired goal.

Patients with diabetes are living longer and are able to live full productive lives, but their paths are by no means easy. Maintenance of blood glucose levels, blood pressures, and lipids are a constant battle. When juggled with busy schedules, this can at times be overwhelming. Further fears of blindness, kidney disease and amputation remain definite prospects, especially for those whose control of systemic conditions is less than optimal. Genetics obviously also plays a role, but this is still not clearly understood. In this book, we review areas under investigation to help us better screen, predict, and understand some mechanisms relating to development of DR. Progress has been made, but much work remains because current treatments are available only near the endpoints of DR. Innovative and effective advances allowing the early detection and intervention of DR are especially relevant and urgently needed.

Author details

Jeffery G. Grigsby[1,2,3] and Andrew T.C. Tsin[4*]

*Address all correspondence to: andrew.tsin@utsa.edu

1 Vision Health Specialties, Midland, Texas, USA

2 College of Optometry, University of Houston, Houston, Texas, USA

3 Texas Tech University Health Science Center, Midland, Texas, USA

4 Department of Biomedical Sciences, University of Texas Rio Grande Valley, School of Medicine, Edinburg, Texas, USA

Section 2

Early Events in Diabetic Retinopathy

Chapter 2

Potential Imaging Biomarkers in the Development and Progression of Diabetic Retinopathy

Julia Hafner, Sonja Karst and Ursula Schmidt-Erfurth

Additional information is available at the end of the chapter

http://dx.doi.org/10.5772/intechopen.71747

Abstract

Diabetic retinopathy (DR) is the most prevalent microvascular complication of diabetes and a leading cause of preventable blindness in the working-age population. However, due to a lack of suitable biomarkers, its prediction in asymptomatic patients is insufficient. Currently, DR is diagnosed at a stage when typical morphologic lesions become fundoscopically visible. Yet, chronically elevated blood glucose levels lead to characteristic alterations in retinal vessel caliber, blood flow, oxygen saturation, and the capillary network, which precede DR lesions. Furthermore, emerging evidence suggests that retinal neurodegenerative changes occur early in diabetes, initiating a disintegration of the retinal neurovascular unit prior to the appearance of microvasculopathy in DR. This chapter will discuss recent research achievements toward understanding the complexities of DR pathophysiology. It will focus on the nomination of potential imaging biomarkers for the prediction of DR development and progression using innovative structural, functional, and metabolic imaging techniques, including optical coherence tomography angiography (OCTA), retinal oximetry, ultra-wide field FA, and corneal confocal microscopy (CCM). Validation of these biomarkers would allow the identification of patients at high risk of developing DR and might initiate a swift move to early diagnosis and individualized care.

Keywords: diabetic retinopathy, biomarker, retinal blood flow, retinal oxygen saturation, retinal neurodegeneration, corneal confocal microscopy, ultra-wide field imaging, disorganization of the inner retinal layers, imaging, OCT, OCTA

1. Introduction: the role of biomarkers in disease prediction

The prevalence of diabetes mellitus is increasing worldwide. The International Diabetes Federation estimated that 415 million people had diabetes in 2015, 90% of whom were diagnosed with type 2 diabetes. With these trends continuing, 642 million patients with diabetes are expected by 2040 [1].

Patients with diabetes are at substantially increased risk of developing complications. In light of the cost of interventions implemented throughout the natural history of these complications, diabetes constitutes a tremendous clinical and public health burden that exceeds the resources of healthcare systems even in the most affluent countries. The International Diabetes Federation has reported that most countries spent 5–20% of their total healthcare budget on diabetes in 2015, which amounted to 673 billion US dollars in health expenditure worldwide. This figure is expected to increase to about 802 billion US dollars by 2040 [1].

The complications of diabetes are commonly divided into macrovascular complications including myocardial infarction, heart failure, and stroke, and microvascular complications including diabetic nephropathy, neuropathy, and retinopathy. Diabetic retinopathy (DR) is the most common microvascular complication of diabetes. The incidence of DR increases with the duration of diabetes. After 20 years, nearly all patients with type 1 diabetes and more than 60% of those with type 2 diabetes will develop signs of DR [2].

Current treatment guidelines target proliferative disease and macular edema, two sight threatening complications. The most common approaches are intravitreal injections of vascular endothelial growth factor (VEGF)-inhibiting agents or corticosteroids, laser treatments, and surgical interventions. These treatments are often sight saving, but are invasive and cost-prohibitive. Therefore, we need to shift our focus to targeting upstream events at earlier stages of non-proliferative DR (NPDR).

The major health economic burden caused by the increasing number of patients diagnosed with diabetes raises the need to identify patients at high risk of developing DR and sight threatening complications. Reliable biomarkers that help to predict the development and progression of the disease have to be defined.

A biomarker is traditionally defined as "a characteristic that is objectively measured and evaluated as an indicator of normal biological processes, pathogenic processes, or pharmacological responses to a therapeutic intervention" [3]. In order to be useful in the prevention of DR, a biomarker should (1) non-invasively detect early preclinical disease before the first clinical signs of the disease appear, (2) be causally linked or be an indicator of a causal mechanism that leads to the development of the disease, and (3) be consistently and strongly associated with the disease [3, 4]. Suitable biomarkers should identify patients at low risk to defer DR screening intervals facilitating cost-effective management and optimized resource allocation. Furthermore, biomarkers should help to predict the progression of DR to the vision-threatening stage, and may forecast the response to different treatment modalities, facilitating individualized care [5]. Important factors for valid biomarkers are reproducibility and validity in different populations. Furthermore, their measurements must be quick, cost-effective, and applicable in daily clinical decision-making [5].

To date, many serum variables have been proposed to be associated with DR incidence and progression. According to the Diabetes Control and Complications Trial (DCCT), a median glycated hemoglobin (HbA1c) of 7.2% reduced DR incidence by 76% in patients

http://dx.doi.org/10.5772/intechopen.71747

with type 1 diabetes, and DR progression by 54% over a period of 6.5 years [6, 7]. Patients with type 2 diabetes had a 25% reduction of DR with good glycemic control [8]. Even though HbA1c remains the most widely accepted biomarker nowadays [5], the "Joslin 50-Year Medalist Study," which focused on the identification of endogenous protective factors in patients with a diabetes duration of at least 50 years (therefore named "Medalists") showed that longitudinal glycemic control was unrelated to diabetic complications. However, the presence of specific advanced glycation end products (AGEs) (plasma carboxyethyl-lysine and pentosidine) was strongly associated with the development of diabetic vasculopathy complications [9].

Cytokines from aqueous humor or vitreous sample have also been considered in the search for a DR biomarker. Increased levels of vascular endothelial growth factor (VEGF), platelet-derived growth factor (PDGF), transforming growth factor beta (TGF-β), and nitric oxide (NO) are commonly found in DR. However, these biomarkers can only be assessed using invasive methods. As tears are more accessible than serum and intraocular fluids (i.e., vitreous or aqueous humor), research has also started to focus on the presence of potential markers in this body fluid. Candidate biomarkers in tear fluid include nerve growth factor (NGF), lipocalin-1, lactotransferrin, lysozyme C, lacritin, lipophilin A, immunoglobulin lambda chain, heat shock protein 27 (HSP 27), and tumor necrosis factor-α (TNF-α) [10].

Ocular imaging biomarkers would offer the advantage of gaining an insight in the actual pathologic evolution of DR non-invasively. The most important candidates for such biomarkers will be discussed in the following chapter.

2. Microvascular changes in diabetic retinopathy

2.1. Retinal vessel caliber

Diabetic retinopathy is diagnosed clinically by the presence of microaneurysms and small hemorrhages visualized during fundoscopy. Assessing the presence and number of microaneurysms as well as their rate of formation and disappearance has been suggested to be an appropriate marker of retinal vascular damage and therefore DR progression [11]. However, there are microvascular changes that have been shown to antecede fundoscopically visible lesions of DR including microaneurysms.

Within the last decades and with the implementation of specialized computer software systems, grading of retinal vessel diameters to document generalized vessel narrowing or widening has become increasingly sophisticated, objective, and reliable. Multiple population-based studies have used these systems to calculate retinal vascular caliber in terms of the central retinal artery and vein equivalent (CRAE, CRVE), which summarizes the average diameter of the internal lumen of the vessel, reflecting the visualized erythrocyte column [12]. In sum, the results of these studies provide evidence for an association between larger venular caliber and DR in patients with type 1 [11, 13] as well as type 2 diabetes [14, 15], therefore being consistent with clinical experience. However, reported findings on arteriolar caliber remain contradictory.

The population-based Multi-Ethnic Study of Atherosclerosis (MESA) study showed that arteriolar calibers are dilated in patients with diabetes [13], whereas other researchers claim that arteries tend to constrict in diabetes [14, 16].

The discrepancy between results of different studies may be due to differences between the study cohorts in demographic (e.g., distribution in age) and metabolic traits including blood glucose levels, duration of diabetes, and cardiovascular risk factors (such as hypertension/hyperlipidemia) as well as differences in sample size, follow-up period, and the methods applied. Before retinal vascular caliber assessment can be used as a biomarker in clinical practice, age-, sex-, body size-, and blood pressure-specific normative data are required.

2.2. Autoregulation of retinal vessel diameter

Besides a "static" measurement of retinal vessel diameter, "dynamic" changes in the diabetic retinal vasculature can be assessed too. The potential for an efficient diameter change in order to adjust blood flow according to changes in arterial blood pressure (pressure autoregulation) and retinal metabolism (metabolic autoregulation) is reduced in the early stages of DR [17]. Vasoactive molecules activate pericytes and smooth muscle cells to regulate the capillary diameter [18]. A dysfunction in pressure autoregulation of retinal arterioles implies that changes in the arterial blood pressure are directly transmitted to the retinal microcirculation [19]. The fact that pressure autoregulation decreases with increasing severity of DR highlights the destructive effect of arterial hypertension on the retinal microcirculation [17, 20].

Luminance flicker stimulation is an example to test the capability of retinal vessels to adapt perfusion to changes in retinal metabolism. Exposure to flickering light stimulates retinal neuronal cells to release local vasodilating metabolites, most importantly nitric oxide [21], which consequently leads to retinal vasodilatation. This results in an increase in retinal blood flow in healthy individuals [22]. Several studies have reported that the flicker light-induced vasodilation is reduced in patients with diabetes [17, 23, 24] and even in patients with prediabetes [25], being equivalent in magnitude to patients with manifest diabetes. Thus, monitoring retinal vascular reactivity may provide an early marker of autoregulation and endothelial dysfunction in the retinal microcirculation that clinicians could follow non-invasively.

2.3. Retinal blood flow

Besides measurement of retinal vessel caliber, numerous other techniques such as laser Doppler velocimetry, laser Doppler flowmetry (LDF), fluorescein angiography (FA), color Doppler, and Doppler optical coherence tomography (OCT) imaging have been proposed for quantifying retinal blood flow in patients with diabetes [26–30]. Contradicting results concerning retinal blood flow have been published. This may reflect the complexities of the pathological alterations that occur in the diabetic retina.

Most studies suggest that in patients without or with mild non-proliferative DR (NPDR), retinal blood flow is reduced [26, 27]. Evidence from animal studies in streptozotocin-treated rats also suggests decreased retinal blood flow in the very early stages of DR [31]. In more severe stages of NPDR, research has provided evidence that retinal blood flow increases above normal levels [28–30], which may arise from the increased demand caused by tissue hypoxia due to capillary basement membrane thickening and capillary occlusion [29, 32]. In proliferative disease, retinal blood flow is decreased again as measured with different techniques: Blair et al. used the dye dilution technique to measure the mean circulation time (MCT) calculated as the difference between the mean venous and arterial retinal passage times, which turned out to be statistically significantly longer in the eyes with proliferative DR (PDR) than in healthy eyes or eyes with NPDR [33]. Laser Doppler flowmetry (LDF), which measures blood flow at the optic nerve head (ONH), and color Doppler imaging, also showed a greater reduction in total retinal blood flow in patients with PDR than in patients with NPDR or healthy individuals [34, 35]. Recently, several groups have demonstrated the potential of Doppler OCT for assessing retinal blood flow in the diabetic eye. Doppler OCT can also detect volumetric blood flow and provide information about the structural anatomy. As shown with the techniques mentioned above, eyes with PDR had statistically significantly decreased retinal blood flow compared with normal eyes [36], especially those that had been treated with panretinal photocoagulation [28, 37, 38]. However, acute elevations in blood glucose can still trigger an increase in blood flow [26]. This finding suggests that the chronic hyperglycemic state in diabetes mellitus is associated with a reduction in retinal blood flow, but the retina still is able to respond to increased metabolic rates associated with acutely raised blood glucose by increasing retinal blood flow.

2.4. The capillary network

The structure of the retinal capillary network is unique. It has to feed one of the highest metabolically active tissues while limiting the extent of the vascular beds to a minimum in order to prevent optical interference to the photoreceptors [39]. The inner retina is perfused by four interconnected capillary plexi that include the peripapillary capillary plexus which is found in the retinal nerve fiber layer (RNFL) adjacent to the optic nerve head (ONH), the superficial capillary plexus in the ganglion cell layer (GCL), as well as an intermediate (ICP) and a deep capillary plexus (DCP), which are located at the two borders of the inner nuclear layer (INL) [40]. Currently most segmentation algorithms display the ICP and DCP as one capillary layer. The three vascular layers unite in the center of the macula to form a terminal capillary ring surrounding the foveal avascular zone (FAZ). The outer retina and the photoreceptors are dependent on blood supplied by diffusion from the choriocapillaris. The early changes in capillary architecture and perfusion in patients with diabetes have not yet been definitely established, as assessing the human retinal microvasculature *in vivo* is very difficult due to its small size and low optical contrast.

FA, introduced in 1961, has been the gold standard imaging technique for assessing the retinal capillary network [41]. The value of this imaging modality is undeniable, but so are its limitations. First, dye leakage and the superimposition of capillary beds from the different retinal layers into a single two-dimensional image hinder a proper differentiation between the superficial and deep capillary plexi [42]. Furthermore, FA is a time-consuming and invasive technique which does not render it optimal for DR screening or frequent longitudinal evaluation. In addition, intravenous fluorescein dye injections can occasionally cause adverse side effects, nausea/vomiting, urticaria and rarely, but critically, anaphylactic reactions in healthy people [43].

Optical coherence tomography angiography (OCTA) is a further advance in retinal microvascular evaluation and may represent a significant breakthrough in ophthalmic imaging, especially in diabetes care. Intravenous injection of extrinsic fluorescent dye is no longer required with this technology, but the perfused capillary architecture is non-invasively visualized with erythrocyte motion as an intrinsic contrast. A recent study has demonstrated that shorter acquisition times and a higher number of motion artifact-free images can be achieved using swept source technology [42].

Several features of early disruption of microvascular perfusion in the development and progression of DR have already been investigated and objectively quantified using OCTA. Diabetic macular ischemia, clinically defined as an enlargement and disruption of the foveal avascular zone (FAZ) and capillary dropout in adjacent parafoveal areas [44], is thought to have predictive potential for DR progression [45]. The considerable inter-subject variability in FAZ size even in healthy people and the large overlap in FAZ size between healthy individuals and patients with diabetes have to be considered though [46]. Hence, FAZ size alone was suggested to be a poor diagnostic variable [47], and qualitative FAZ assessment (e.g., with FAZ outline and regularity) may constitute a more reliable biomarker for the ischemic state of the macula in the diagnosis of DR, either complementary to or in place of a quantitative assessment [48].

OCTA is also reproducible for the measurement of vessel density in healthy eyes and eyes with DR. Compared with a healthy control group, patients with diabetes but without DR were shown to feature reduced parafoveal and perifoveal vessel density, and intercapillary areas increase as DR progresses [47, 49, 50]. A more consistent and severe decrease in vessel density has been observed in the superficial capillary network than in the deep plexus in most studies [51, 52]. Accordingly, mean vessel density in the superficial retinal layer, being highly inversely correlated to best-corrected visual acuity (BCVA), has already been proposed to be the best marker for a reliable differentiation between healthy eyes and those with DR [53]. Similarly, the total avascular area in the central 5.5-mm-diameter area was shown to distinguish eyes with DR from control eyes with 100% sensitivity and specificity. It was, therefore, suggested that total avascular area may be an excellent biomarker in the diagnosis of DR [47].

Compared with FA, where the edges of non-perfused areas appear fuzzy or cannot be detected at all, OCT angiograms clearly delimit the border between sparse-capillary areas and dense-capillary areas in most cases [52, 54]. Choi et al. also found impairment of flow in the choriocapillaris at all stages of DR, supporting the concept that choriocapillaris alterations may play a role in the pathogenesis of DR [55].

OCTA color-coded perfusion density mapping enhances areas of low capillary perfusion density in the SCP, DCP and the choriocapillaris in patients with diabetes. Additional trend analysis has shown a statistically significant decrease in capillary perfusion density values as DR progressed [56].

OCTA techniques have also been used to study the development and progression, as well as the treatment response of clinically visible signs of DR. Microaneurysms can be identified in OCTA, but with a significantly lower sensitivity compared with conventional FA [52]. Nevertheless, OCTA provides additional information about their originating capillary plexus. Significantly, more microaneurysms were found in the intermediate/deep capillary plexus than in the superficial one [54, 57]. Additionally, it has been proposed that OCTA is more useful to evaluate clinically active microaneurysms, which are a major cause of diabetic macular edema (DME) [58]. Intraretinal microvascular abnormalities (IRMA), on the other hand, were well detected by both FA and OCTA [54].

The significance of the individual evaluation of the integrity of the deep capillary plexus, impossible with FA alone, is further supported as macular outer retinal changes on spectral-domain OCT (SD-OCT) correspond to areas of capillary non-perfusion at the level of the DCP in patients with DR. The spectrum of outer retinal alterations encompassed different degrees of thinning of the outer nuclear layer (ONL), disruption of the photoreceptor lines, and focal photoreceptor layer thinning [59].

Diagnosis of retinal neovascularization on FA depends on identifying characteristic pathologic vessels with profuse leakage in late angiographic phases. With OCTA, spots of neovascularization that were not identified with FA were visualized as an abnormal flow signal above the inner limiting membrane, which may further help in the identification of patients requiring treatment [47, 55].

Certainly, there are limitations to the OCTA systems in their current state that have to be acknowledged including the incidence of motion artifacts and the relatively small field of view [41], but these can be improved with future development efforts [60]. In summary, OCTA enables the visualization of early microvascular perfusion abnormalities representing imminent DR development and simultaneous monitoring of the treatment response of pathognomonic lesions of DR. It could therefore provide clinicians and scientists in clinical trials with valuable and reliable biomarkers, using an imaging technology that is safely tolerated by patients.

2.5. Retinal oxygen supply

Capillary non-perfusion and tissue ischemia are well-known hallmarks of diabetic retinopathy. While FA provides information about the anatomic state of retinal vessels, changes in retinal oxygenation reflect metabolic dysfunction. Oxygen saturation (SO2) in retinal vessels is a direct measure of retinal oxygen metabolism [18].

Using retinal oximetry, retinal SO2 can be measured non-invasively in major retinal arterioles and venules. The retinal oximeter records fundus images reflected from the retina at two different wavelengths, one being sensitive to oxygen (600 nm), and one being insensitive to oxygen (570 nm). An inverse linear relation between the optical density ratio measured at the two wavelengths and SO2 is assumed. Retinal oxygen saturation can be presented numerically and as a color saturation map [61]. Low variability as well as high reproducibility and repeatability have been shown for retinal oximetry measurements in healthy individuals and in diseased retinas [62–64]. Furthermore, there have already been a number of approaches to compile normative databases for retinal oximetry measurements in Caucasian [61] and multiethnic populations [65], to set a basis for comparability for future clinical trials. Age is the most important factor that should be accounted for in the interpretation of retinal oximetry measurements. Beside age and ethnicity, other demographic factors do not seem to influence retinal oximetry results markedly [61, 65, 66]. Additionally, no statistically significant difference in SO2 levels between patients with type 1 and type 2 diabetes could be observed [61].

Oxygen saturation levels in retinal vessels seem to steadily increase with progressing severity of DR, even if it is not fully elucidated if both, arterioles and venules [67, 68], or solely venules are affected by this increase [69]. Compared with healthy individuals, the change in SO2 levels only becomes statistically significant at more advanced stages of severe NPDR or PDR. Some investigators support the concept that in earlier stages of DR, increased levels of SO2 are detected in retinal venules only, which stands for a decreasing oxygen extraction in these patients, whereas in patients with PDR, SO2 levels are also increased in retinal arterioles, resulting in unchanged levels of oxygen extraction [70].

The metabolic results reflected by retinal oximetry also seem to correlate with the extent of retinal ischemia measured in FA [67].

At first, the findings of increased oxygen saturation levels in patients with diabetes with or without DR seem to conflict with the traditional concept of DR being an ischemic disease. However, this observation can be explained by at least three mechanisms: (1) capillary non-perfusion and shunting (2) thickening of the basement membrane of capillary vessel walls, and (3) greater affinity of hemoglobin for oxygen [71]. Capillary non-perfusion in conjunction with the formation of shunt vessel is already known from histologic studies in the diabetic retina. In capillary shunting, while some vessels dilate, others constrict, leading to blood flow bypassing parts of the capillary network. Blood is then transported faster through these dilated preferential channels, resulting in a shortened arterio-venous passage time and therefore a reduced oxygen extraction time [72]. Further, with thickening of the capillary basement membranes, inevitably, oxygen diffusion from the blood to the retinal tissue is hindered as the transport distance increases [73]. All these mechanisms lead to a maldistribution of oxygen. Oxygen cannot be delivered to the retinal cells in these ischemic areas, which makes venular blood relatively hyperoxic and retinal tissue relatively hypoxic. As a compensatory response, oxygen demand will increase, and more blood will be directed to the tissue. Therefore, oxygenation in arterioles increases too [68].

Intraocular injections of substances inhibiting the production of vascular endothelial growth factor (VEGF), as well as laser treatment and vitrectomy are therapeutic for complications in advanced DR and all of them influence retinal oxygen metabolism.

The vitreous cavities of patients with PDR who have undergone vitrectomy have lower oxygen tension than those who do not have diabetes [74]. Anti-VEGF injections can reduce diabetic macular edema and retinal neovascularization leading to a gain in visual acuity in patients with diabetic maculopathy and/or PDR. The introduction of this treatment modality has considerably improved the visual rehabilitation for patients with DR, but still, some

http://dx.doi.org/10.5772/intechopen.71747

patients respond better to the treatment than others. Interestingly, a recent study indicates that together with arterial blood pressure, SO2 in retinal arterioles may predict visual acuity and central retinal thickness (CRT) in patients with diabetic macular edema after anti-VEGF treatment [75]. Retinal laser treatment destroys retinal tissue and therefore reduces oxygen consumption in treated retinal areas, which in turn reduces hypoxia and the subsequent production of VEGF [76]. The effects of this treatment can be detected with retinal oximetry. A slight increase in SO2 in retinal venules and unchanged SO2 in retinal arterioles was measured immediately after treatment in patients with diabetic maculopathy and patients with PDR, resulting in reduced oxygen extraction. Three months after treatment, arteriolar and venular SO2 were both increased, but arteriovenous SO2 difference was unchanged compared with pretreatment levels [77]. A more recent study in patients with treatment-naive PDR suggested that pre-laser retinal SO2 was not able to predict immediate post-treatment activity of neovascularization, but post-treatment changes in SO2 were closely linked to disease activity 3 months after photocoagulation. Each 1% increase in retinal venular SO2 was independently associated with a 30% higher risk of increased PDR activity despite laser treatment. This implies that if photocoagulation is successfully performed, the amount of the hypoxic retinal tissue is decreased. In the adjacent vital retinal tissue, oxygen is extracted efficiently from retinal arteries, which lowers the venous SO2 and the arteriovenous SO2 levels [78]. Therefore, investigation of oxygen supply may be a potential non-invasive marker of angiogenic disease activity in the monitoring of the treatment response in DR. Prospective studies are under way to further validate retinal oximetry as a biomarker in DR.

3. The identification of lesions in the retinal periphery

Increasing evidence from research suggests that the first lesions in DR develop in the periphery of the retina and that these lesions are potentially associated with DR progression [79, 80]. The gold standard for determining the severity of DR is the extended modified Airlie House classification, which was first used in the Early Treatment Diabetic Retinopathy Study (ETDRS) in 1991 [81]. This rigorously standardized grading scale comprises 13 distinct levels, ranging from the absence of DR to the most severe manifestations of the disease localized in the central posterior 90° of the retina, representing approximately 30% of the entire retinal surface. The ETDRS grading scale is an established measure of disease activity and predictive of the risk of DR progression and visual loss over time [82]. However, due to imaging limitations, a systematic assessment of the retinal periphery was not feasible when the original ETDRS criteria were created. Therefore, the presence of pathologic features outside the 7-fields of ETDRS photography was not accounted for in this grading scale. With the advent of commercially available high-resolution ultrawide-field (UWF) scanning laser ophthalmoscopes, peripheral retinal lesions within and outside the area of the 7-standard ETDRS fields can now be evaluated [83]. Instead of 30° captured by a single ETDRS photo, these UWF imaging systems cover up to 200° in a single image, representing approximately 82% of the retinal area. Combining low-powered green (532 nm) and red (633 nm) laser light, a composite color image with a resolution of 14 μm can be acquired in just a quarter of a second. The high-resolution scanning laser ophthalmoscopy UWF technique allows improved imaging through media opacities such as cataracts, and images can even be acquired without pupillary mydriasis.

There are a number of examples in the literature showing that UWF imaging is comparable to conventional retinal imaging techniques for DR grading. In these studies, images were evaluated for the presence of predominantly peripheral lesions (PPLs), defined as lesions with more than 50% of the lesion located outside one of the ETDRS fields. Compared with eyes without PPL, it is estimated that eyes with PPL at baseline have a 3.2-fold increased risk of a 2-step or more DR progression and a 4.7-fold increased risk for progression to PDR over 4 years, independent of baseline DR severity and HbA1c levels [84].

Identification of DR lesions with non-mydriatic UWF imaging has been compared with standard non-mydriatic multifield fundus photography (NMFP) in large population-based DR teleophthalmology programs. Determining the risk for DR progression associated with an individual's retinal findings in imaging is fundamental in such programs for appropriate risk assessment as well as timing of screening intervals. Ungradable images generally result in referral for comprehensive eye examination because the severity of DR cannot be ascertained. The efficiency of DR teleophthalmology programs could be improved by reducing the unnecessary referrals due to ungradable images, which would lead to considerable savings in logistical complexities, travel arrangements, and time burdens for patients and the healthcare system [83]. UWF imaging can reduce the ungradable image rate by 71% and image evaluation time by 28% compared with NMFP [85]. UWF imaging additionally resulted in a more severe DR level in 9–15% of eyes [84, 86]. Non-mydriatic UWF images were shown to compare favorably with dilated ETDRS photography in determining DR severity, and discrepancies between ETDRS and UWF images were found to be mostly attributable to hemorrhages or microaneurysms [83, 87]. Silva et al. suggested that approximately one third of lesions including hemorrhages, microaneurysms, IRMA, and neovascularization were found predominantly outside the ETDRS fields, being more frequent in temporal than nasal fields [83]. Furthermore, UWF imaging substantially increases the identification of peripheral non-diabetic lesions such as lattice and other retinal degenerations, retinal tears and holes, and choroidal lesions [88]. The utility of UWF imaging has also been demonstrated in comparison with conventional slit-lamp biomicroscopy in a "real-life" clinical setting [89], and in comparison with the gold standard dilated fundus examination with scleral indentation, where Optomap showed high specificity and moderate sensitivity for lesions posterior to the equator, but low sensitivity for lesions anterior to the equator [90]. It was even proposed that assessing of UWF combined with OCT images allows more eyes with higher grades of DR to be detected than in a clinical examination alone or combined with imaging in a clinical setting [91].

The ETDRS extensively evaluated FA but did not provide evidence for a substantially improved ability to predict subsequent DR progression applying this technique. However, due to the limited field of view, traditional FA may miss major areas of peripheral capillary non-perfusion and neovascularization. The advent of UWF FA has provided the opportunity to visualize both the central and peripheral retina in a single examination [92]. Sim et al.

evaluated the association between peripheral retinal ischemia of UWF FA images and central ischemia in DR, and observed a moderate correlation between the peripheral ischemic index and FAZ area, as well as peripheral leakage index and FAZ area in eyes which have not been treated with laser yet [44]. Similarly, 3.9 times more non-perfusion, 1.9 times more neovascularization, and 3.8 times more panretinal photocoagulation scars could be detected in UWF FA compared with the 7-standard field ETDRS images [93]. An increase in retinal non-perfusion was associated with worsening DR [94]. As peripheral non-perfusion probably underlies the development of PPL [80], the identification of PPL may be a potential surrogate marker for estimating the location and extent of peripheral non-perfusion [94].

Current study results assessing the value of UWF FA in eyes with diabetic macular edema (DME) are still contradictory [28, 93, 94].

Besides the paramount advantages of incorporating UWF imaging into the diagnosis and management of DR, certain limitations including low portability and the need for extensive imager training to obtain high quality images must be acknowledged [95]. UWF imaging systems are still expensive but their cost is likely to decrease over time with further technological innovations and market competitions.

In summary, peripheral lesions identified in UWF imaging may substantially alter the risk of DR onset, progression and outcome. Currently a new DR severity grading scale will be established combining clinical with imaging information from UWF photographs and angiograms. A large longitudinal multicenter study sponsored by the Diabetic Retinopathy Clinical Research Network (DRCR.net) has been designed to assess the relation between baseline variables on UWF color fundus photographs and UWF FA with long-term DR outcomes [95].

4. Disorganization of the retinal inner layers for diabetic macular edema prediction

Diabetic macular edema (DME) is one of the most vision-threatening manifestations of DR, affecting almost 30% of patients with a duration of diabetes mellitus of more than 20 years [96].

Elevated levels of vascular endothelial growth factor (VEGF) are a major contributor to retinal microvascular dysfunction and the development of DME. VEGF interferes with tight junctions of the vascular endothelium, leading to a breakdown of the blood retinal barrier and consequently leakage into the retinal tissue [97]. Therefore, repetitive intraocular injections of anti-VEGF agents are a first-line therapy among the currently available treatments for DME. These injections have demonstrated efficiency in reducing macular thickness and improving best-corrected visual acuity (BCVA) [98]. However, while beneficial for some patients, others do not respond to intraocular drug injections. Furthermore, the resolution of DME may not be followed by a recovery in visual function. To date, no reliable methods exist to determine which individuals with DME will or will not respond to available treatments. The implementation of predictive biomarkers would guarantee an efficient therapeutic selection to identify patients with a limited prognosis of visual recovery despite ongoing therapeutic actions, where early visual disability support instead of burdensome treatment schedules may be warranted. SD-OCT provides high-resolution imaging of the retinal structure and allows insight into the pathogenesis of DME *in vivo*. Central retinal thickness (CRT) measured with OCT is commonly used in the evaluation and management of DME. However, CRT only explains 27% of the variation in visual acuity [99]. Various other OCT measures have been studied, but none of these measures has been consistently demonstrated to account for visual outcomes in patients with DME, and most of these studies were conducted retrospectively in mixed treatment cohorts. Examples of these measures include the integrity of the ellipsoid zone (EZ) (formerly described as the inner segment/outer segment photoreceptor junction) [100, 101], the integrity of the external limiting membrane [101, 102], the visibility of the cone outer segment tips (COST) [103], as well as the presence of subretinal fluid [104] and hyperreflective foci [105, 106].

Furthermore, intraretinal cystoid fluid has been named as a predictor of poor response to anti-VEGF treatment in a prospective study [101], as well as in two post hoc analyses [107, 108] in large datasets of patients with DME using a machine-learning approach. Recently, disorganization of the retinal inner layers (DRIL) has been suggested to be a valid predictive biomarker for visual outcomes in patients with DME. DRIL was defined as the inability to distinguish boundaries between any two of the inner retinal layers (including the ganglion cell-inner plexiform layer (GCIPL) complex, the inner nuclear layer, and the outer plexiform layer) in >50% of the foveal 1-mm zone [103]. DRIL in the central millimeter is strongly associated with visual acuity in eyes with center-involving DME. Resolving DRIL seemed to be a good indicator of subsequent visual improvement [109]. In addition, the presence and extent of DRIL before treatment are correlated with BCVA outcomes to anti-VEGF therapy after the loading dose of ranibizumab in treatment naive patients with DME [101]. Similarly, patients with DME showed gain in visual acuity if DRIL resolved compared with non-resolvers, whose visual acuity worsened. This correlation between DRIL and visual acuity could not be substantiated for eyes with macular edema due to other causes [110]. Additionally, it is well known that approximately 55% of patients with DME have co-existent macular capillary non-perfusion [111], which may be masked angiographically by leakage from the edema. Macular capillary non-perfusion hinders efficient transport of oxygen and nutrients to the inner retinal layers, which in turn compromises inner retinal integrity and may therefore lead to the appearance of DRIL in OCT scans. This concept has been substantiated by a recent study reporting 84.4% sensitivity and 100% specificity of DRIL in detecting angiographic evidence of capillary non-perfusion in the macula [112].

The exact mechanisms of DRIL affecting VA have yet to be determined, but their correlation in eyes with DME is plausible as DRIL may represent an interruption in anatomic structures within these inner retinal layers including axons and nuclei of bipolar, amacrine, and/or horizontal cells, and therefore a disruption in the visual pathway from photoreceptors to retinal ganglion cells.

These data suggest that DRIL is a robust biomarker of visual acuity in eyes with present or resolved DME, correlating better with visual acuity than other OCT measures including CRT. Future multicenter longitudinal studies have to validate the predictive potential of DRIL by prospectively collecting data on the visual outcome of patients with DME, with additional studies to clarify the histologic equivalent accompanying the appearance of DRIL in SD-OCT [103].

5. Diabetic retinopathy as a neurodegenerative disease

5.1. The neurovascular unit

Fundoscopic clinical examination of patients with DR reveals pathognomonic features including hard exudates, hemorrhages, microaneurysms, and cotton wool spots. However, it does not reveal the complex organization of the neurosensory retina. Similar to other tissues throughout the central nervous system, neurons, glia, microglia, and blood vessels are organized into neurovascular units that work interdependently in close coordination in the retina [113].

The complex interconnections in the neurovascular unit prompted early anatomists to call this tissue the retina, literally a network of cells [114]. The capillary networks of the inner retina are in close contact with neurons of the inner nuclear and ganglion cell layer. These capillaries consist of a basal lamina with a single layer of adherent endothelial cells surrounded by pericytes, glial, and microglial cells on the external surface. Microglia interact directly with retinal pericytes and are intimately associated with retinal neurons [115].

This intimate physical contact and functional integration are essential for vision and facilitate physiologic adaptation in response to varying conditions. Neuronal activity evokes localized reactions including vasodilation and increased blood flow to meet the energy demands of neuronal signal transduction and transmission [114]. In addition to the coordination of metabolic demand, close signaling interdependence manifests itself in the blood-retinal barrier, which controls the flux of fluids and metabolites into the retinal tissue [116].

The diabetic environment causes the neurovascular unit to disintegrate both in early and late DR with the physiology of the neurovascular unit being similarly altered as it is in diseases of the brain such as stroke [117], Alzheimer's, and Parkinson's diseases [118]. Although DR has traditionally been considered merely a microvascular diabetic complication, recent studies support the concept that retinal neurodegeneration precedes and contributes to the formation of microvascular abnormalities in DR. These findings suggest that DR should at least be considered a combined neuro-vascular degeneration [113].

5.2. Retinal neurodegeneration

Signs of neurodegeneration were not visible in fundus examination in the era of the ETDRS. Therefore, these changes did not contribute to the characterization or diagnosis of the disease. However, retinal neurodegeneration has widely been accepted as part of DR over the last decades.

These abnormalities in retinal neural tissue lead to well-studied functional changes that typically precede the clinical diagnosis of DR, and in some cases occur even prior to the diagnosis of diabetes. Neurofunctional impairment becomes apparent as a dysfunction in dark adaptation [119], abnormal contrast sensitivity [120], and altered microperimetry [105], as well as electroretinogram (ERG) results. The electroretinogram (ERG) is one of the most effective diagnostic tools in this context, with the oscillatory potential implicit time being the most consistent and widely reported aspect of the ERG that changes early in DR [121]. A delay in implicit time in multifocal ERG (mfERG) has been shown to be highly predictive (86% sensitivity and 84% specificity) of new retinopathy development at specific locations over 3 years in patients with early stages of DR at baseline [122, 123]. The European Consortium for the Early Treatment of Diabetic Retinopathy (EUROCONDOR) trial currently tests mfERG for its use and potential in DR prediction. However, while ERG is a very sensitive technique to detect neurofunctional deficits, it is also a quite burdensome and time-consuming examination.

Anatomical evaluation of retinal neurodegeneration has become possible with the implementation of SD-OCT. In OCT, the most useful measure for identifying diabetes-induced neurodegeneration is the thickness-reduction of the retinal nerve fiber layer (RNFL) and the ganglion cell complex, consisting of the ganglion cell layer (GCL) and the inner plexiform layer (IPL). Retinal ganglion cells (RGCs) are the retinal neurons in which the apoptotic process related to diabetes is first detected [124]. An impaired integrity of these cells compromises information processing and the transmission of visual signals to the brain. The damage primarily affects the RGC's nuclei and dendrites, as shown by a diffuse thinning of the combined retinal ganglion cell-inner plexiform layer (GCIPL). Secondarily, their axons are affected too, as indicated by a reduction of the retinal nerve fiber layer (RNFL) thickness [125]. A significant thinning of the GCIPL complex alone [126] or in combination with thinning of the RNFL has already been shown in patients with type 1 diabetes even without any fundoscopically manifest signs of DR [127, 128]. A longitudinal analysis in patients with type 1 diabetes depicted an average progressive thickness loss of 0.25 μm/year and 0.29 μm/year in the RNFL and the GCL + IPL, respectively, over a 4-year follow-up period in patients with no or minimal DR, independent of age, sex and even Hb1Ac. Intriguingly, the extent of thickness loss was similar to that of patients with severe glaucoma [129]. Research results are also consistent in finding reduced RNFL and GCIPL thicknesses in patients with type 2 diabetes [130–132].

Further, relation between structural signs of diabetic retinal neurodegeneration and functional deficits has been investigated thoroughly. Reduced GCIPL complex thickness has been shown to significantly correlate with impaired visual function assessed by contrast sensitivity and pattern ERG amplitudes in patients with diabetes without DR [131]. In patients with type 1 diabetes and no or minimal DR, GCL thickness was an important predictor of loss of macular visual function measured by the Rarebit perimetry [133].

Research has also started to focus on the temporal and causal relationship of neurogenic and vascular changes in DR. Preliminary results of the EUROCONDOR study suggest that in patients with no or mild DR, retinal vessel caliber is independently associated with structural changes of the neuroretina. Specifically, CRAE was statistically significantly associated with macular GCL thickness and CRVE with RNFL thickness at the optic disc [134]. An association of venular dilatation and thinning of the RNFL along with deficits in the ERG was detected in adolescents with type 2 diabetes, showing that the structural changes are accompanied by early vascular dysfunction [135].

The mechanisms behind this neurodegeneration are not completely clear. Increased apoptosis in neuronal tissue may be caused by chronic hyperglycemia, when neuronal cells experience up to 4-fold increase in glucose uptake. If hyperglycemia is prolonged, nerves are damaged [136]. Additionally, glucose and glutamate accumulation in the extracellular space, increased oxidative stress, inflammation and imbalance in the production of neuroprotective factors are other factors thought to be involved in the development of neurodegeneration in the setting of DR [137]. Apoptosis of the retinal ganglion cells also tends to be accompanied by reactive changes in macroglial cells, known as "reactive gliosis." Apart from astrocytes, the predominant type of macroglia is the Müller cell, which is unique to the retina. One of the most prominent characteristics of reactive gliosis is that Müller cells overexpress glial acidic fibrillary protein (GFAP), which is considered a sensitive indicator of central nervous system injury, and is normally only expressed by retinal astrocytes [138]. Müller cells span the entire retina, surround all blood vessels, and produce molecules that contribute to the modulation of blood flow and vascular permeability. In addition, they are essential for the survival of neurons. Therefore, glial cells, and especially Müller cells, are thought to play a key role in the pathogenesis of both retinal microangiopathy and neurodegeneration. Unfortunately, Müller cells can currently not be imaged *in vivo.*

Because neurons cannot be replaced, DR becomes irreversible with continuous disease progression. The identification of biomarkers that predict the development of neurodegeneration as well as mediators in the cross talk between neurodegeneration and microangiopathy is crucial for the development of new therapeutic strategies in DR. Safe and effective neuroprotective agents could possibly prevent neuronal apoptosis and vision loss but also impede the impairment of neurovascular coupling. Consequently, microvascular impairment and clinically apparent DR could be delayed. Evidence from the numerous studies mentioned above suggests that diabetic retinal neurodegeneration most likely precedes the microvasculopathy of DR. Functional examinations, like mfERG as well as structural evaluation of the inner retinal layers with SD-OCT may permit an early detection of the disease. However, further longitudinal studies are required to clarify the precise temporal relation between neurodegeneration and the microvascular alterations of DR.

5.3. Neurodegeneration outside the retina

Neurodegenerative changes occur outside the retina too. The cornea is one of the most densely innervated structures of the human body. A rich network of sensory nerves, known as the subbasal nerve plexus (SNP), derives from the ophthalmic division of the trigeminal nerve and lies between the corneal epithelium and Bowman's membrane [139]. This layer can be visualized with corneal confocal microscopy (CCM), a highly reproducible [140] in vivo imaging technique that provides diagnostic efficiency comparable to that of intra-epidermal nerve fiber density (IENFD) assessment [141, 142]. IENFD is the current gold standard for evaluating small nerve fiber damage, but is invasive, time-consuming and requires significant laboratory expertise. Evaluation of small fiber neuropathy is essential, as they constitute 70–90% of peripheral nerves and are preferentially involved in the development of diabetic peripheral neuropathy (DPN). DPN affects at least 50% of patients with diabetes mellitus and is the main initiating factor for foot ulceration and subsequent lower extremity amputation [143]. Unfortunately, to date, the guidelines for DPN mainly advocate electrophysiology besides clinical symptom testing, which is sensitive only for the detection of large fiber damage [144]. CCM could potentially serve as a non-invasive, objective biomarker for identifying small fiber damage and making an early diagnosis of DPN. The main changes in SNP morphology detected in patients with diabetes include a decrease in corneal nerve fiber density (CNFD), defined as the total number of major nerves per mm^2; corneal nerve fiber length (CNFL), defined as the total length of all nerve fibers and branches (mm/mm^2); and corneal nerve branch density (CNBD), defined as the number of branches emanating from major nerves per mm^2 [145]. Previous studies have evaluated the relationship between SNP morphology and the development and progression of DR. SNP impairment appears to progress in parallel with DR and could even be demonstrated in patients with diabetes without DR [146–149]. This finding would support the concept that besides neuronal loss in the retina, corneal neurodegeneration might precede the development of visible microangiopathy in DR too.

Even though recent studies indicate that inner retinal layer thinning representing retinal neurodegeneration is associated with DPN, the direct relation between SNP morphology and variables of retinal neurodegeneration has not yet been clarified. Eventually, CCM has the potential to be a surrogate for an early diagnosis of and an early biomarker for DR and DPN that could identify those at risk.

6. Conclusions

Diabetes mellitus is clearly a major health problem in an increasingly aging population worldwide. Diabetic retinopathy is a complex complication of this disease, which is influenced by a range of local and systemic factors. Potential non-invasive biomarkers derived from innovative imaging modalities as introduced above offer precious information about the morphologic as well as functional state of the diabetic retina, which is not detectable on routine clinical examination. These promising biomarkers may allow personalized medicine with treatment schedules tailored to patients' individual needs. Furthermore, as the population principally affected by DR comprises working-age individuals, understanding of the pathophysiology of the disease and developing appropriate therapy are essential to halt decrease in productivity and an increasing need for social support. Besides this significant economic benefit, the final validation of these biomarkers in prospective studies is expected to contribute decisively to the designing of clinical trials to identify new drug candidates that may prevent DR in the initial disease stages. Finally, and most importantly, this could result in a dramatic quality-of-life improvement for patients with diabetes and their families.

Author details

Julia Hafner*, Sonja Karst and Ursula Schmidt-Erfurth

*Address all correspondence to: julia.hafner@meduniwien.ac.at

Department of Ophthalmology and Optometry, Medical University of Vienna, Vienna, Austria

References

[1] Herman WH. The global burden of diabetes: An overview. In: Dagogo-Jack S, editor. Diabetes Mellitus in Developing Countries and Underserved Communities. Cham: Springer International Publishing; 2017. pp. 1-5

[2] Fong DS, Aiello L, Gardner TW, King GL, Blankenship G, Cavallerano JD, et al. Retinopathy in diabetes. Diabetes Care. 2004;**27**(Suppl 1):S84-S87

[3] Steyerberg EW, Pencina MJ, Lingsma HF, Kattan MW, Vickers AJ, Van Calster B. Assessing the incremental value of diagnostic and prognostic markers: A review and illustration. European Journal of Clinical Investigation. 2012;**42**:216-228

[4] Ikram MK, Cheung CY, Lorenzi M, Klein R, Jones TLZ, Wong TY. Retinal vascular caliber as a biomarker for diabetes microvascular complications. Diabetes Care. 2013;**36**: 750-759

[5] Ting DSW, Tan GSW, Agrawal R, Yanagi Y, Sie NM, Wong CW, et al. Optical coherence tomographic angiography in type 2 diabetes and diabetic retinopathy. JAMA Ophthalmology. 2017;**135**:306-312

[6] Lachin JM, Genuth S, Cleary P, Davis MD, Nathan DM. Retinopathy and nephropathy in patients with type 1 diabetes four years after a trial of intensive therapy. The New England Journal of Medicine. 2000;**342**:381-389

[7] Diabetes Control and Complications Trial Research Group. Progression of retinopathy with intensive versus conventional treatment in the Diabetes Control and Complications Trial. Ophthalmology. 1995;**102**:647-661

[8] UK Prospective Diabetes Study (UKPDS) Group. Intensive blood-glucose control with sulphonylureas or insulin compared with conventional treatment and risk of complications in patients with type 2 diabetes (UKPDS 33). Lancet (London, England). 1998;**352**: 837-853

[9] Sun JK, Keenan HA, Cavallerano JD, Asztalos BF, Schaefer EJ, Sell DR, et al. Protection from retinopathy and other complications in patients with type 1 diabetes of extreme duration: The joslin 50-year medalist study. Diabetes Care. 2011;**34**(4):968-974

[10] Hagan S, Martin E, Enriquez-de-Salamanca A. Tear fluid biomarkers in ocular and systemic disease: Potential use for predictive, preventive and personalised medicine. The EPMA Journal. 2016;**7**:15

[11] Klein R, Klein BEK, Moss SE, Wong TY, Hubbard L, Cruickshanks KJ, et al. The relation of retinal vessel caliber to the incidence and progression of diabetic retinopathy: XIX: The Wisconsin epidemiologic study of diabetic retinopathy. (Chicago, IL: 1960). Archives of Ophthalmology. 2004;**122**:76-83

[12] Hubbard LD, Brothers RJ, King WN, Clegg LX, Klein R, Cooper LS, et al. Methods for evaluation of retinal microvascular abnormalities associated with hypertension/sclerosis in the atherosclerosis risk in communities study. Ophthalmology. 1999;**106**:2269-2280

[13] Tien YW, Islam FMA, Klein R, Klein BEK, Cotch MF, Castro C, et al. Retinal vascular caliber, cardiovascular risk factors, and inflammation: The multi-ethnic study of atherosclerosis (MESA). Investigative Ophthalmology and Visual Science. 2006;**47**:2341-2350

[14] Klein R, Klein BEK, Moss SE, Wong TY. Retinal vessel caliber and microvascular and macrovascular disease in type 2 diabetes. XXI: The Wisconsin epidemiologic study of diabetic retinopathy. Ophthalmology. 2007;**114**:1884-1892

[15] Yang X, Deng Y, Gu H, Ren X, Lim A, Snellingen T, et al. Relationship of retinal vascular calibre and diabetic retinopathy in Chinese patients with type 2 diabetes mellitus: the Desheng Diabetic Eye Study. Br J Ophthalmol. 2016 Oct;**100**(10):1359-65. DOI: 10.1136/bjophthalmol-2014-306078. Epub 2016 Jan 28

[16] Dong Y, Lin L, Yan H, Fu Y, Zong Y, Yuan Y, et al. Shifts in retinal vessel diameter and oxygen saturation in Chinese type 2 diabetes mellitus patients. BMC Ophthalmology. 2016;**16**:43

[17] Bek T. Diameter Changes of Retinal Vessels in Diabetic Retinopathy. Curr Diab Rep. 2017 Aug 8;**17**(10):82. DOI: 10.1007/s11892-017-0909-9

[18] Hardarson SH, Harris A, Karlsson RA, Halldorsson GH, Kagemann L, Rechtman E, et al. Automatic retinal oximetry. Investigative Opthalmology and Visual Science. 2006;**47**:5011

[19] Kohner EM, Patel V, Rassam SM. Role of blood flow and impaired autoregulation in the pathogenesis of diabetic retinopathy. Diabetes. 1995;**44**:603-607

[20] Frederiksen CA, Jeppesen P, Knudsen ST, Poulsen PL, Mogensen CE, Bek T. The blood pressure-induced diameter response of retinal arterioles decreases with increasing diabetic maculopathy. Graefe's Archive for Clinical and Experimental Ophthalmology = Albrecht von Graefes Archiv fur klinische und experimentelle Ophthalmologie. 2006;**244**:1255-1261

[21] Schmetterer L, Findl O, Fasching P, Ferber W, Strenn K, Breiteneder H, et al. Nitric oxide and ocular blood flow in patients with IDDM. Diabetes. 1997;**46**:653-658

[22] Michelson G, Patzelt A, Harazny J. Flickering light increases retinal blood flow. Retina (Philadelphia, PA). 2002;**22**:336-343

[23] Garhofer G, Zawinka C, Resch H, Kothy P, Schmetterer L, Dorner GT. Reduced response of retinal vessel diameters to flicker stimulation in patients with diabetes. The British Journal of Ophthalmology. 2004;**88**:887-891

[24] Pemp B, Garhofer G, Weigert G, Karl K, Resch H, Wolzt M, et al. Reduced retinal vessel response to flicker stimulation but not to exogenous nitric oxide in type 1 diabetes. Investigative Ophthalmology and Visual Science. 2009;**50**:4029-4032

[25] Lott MEJ, Slocomb JE, Shivkumar V, Smith B, Quillen D, Gabbay RA, et al. Impaired retinal vasodilator responses in prediabetes and type 2 diabetes. Acta Ophthalmologica. 2013;**91**:1-18

[26] Bursell SE, Clermont AC, Kinsley BT, Simonson DC, Aiello LM, Wolpert HA. Retinal blood flow changes in patients with insulin-dependent diabetes mellitus and no diabetic retinopathy. Investigative Ophthalmology and Visual Science. 1996;**37**:886-897

[27] Nagaoka T, Sato E, Takahashi A, Yokota H, Sogawa K, Yoshida A. Impaired retinal circulation in patients with type 2 diabetes mellitus: Retinal laser Doppler Velocimetry Study. Investigative Ophthalmology and Visual Science. 2010;**51**:6729-6734

[28] Patel V, Rassam S, Newsom R, Wiek J, Kohner E. Retinal blood flow in diabetic retinopathy. British Medical Journal (Clinical Research Edition). 1992;**305**:678-683

[29] Kohner EM, Hamilton AM, Saunders SJ, Sutcliffe BA, Bulpitt CJ. The retinal blood flow in diabetes. Diabetologia. 1975;**11**:27-33

[30] Grunwald JE, Riva CE, Sinclair SH, Brucker AJ, Petrig BL. Laser Doppler velocimetry study of retinal circulation in diabetes mellitus. Archives of Ophthalmology (Chicago, IL: 1960). 1986;**104**:991-996

[31] Takagi C, Bursell SE, Lin YW, Takagi H, Duh E, Jiang Z, et al. Regulation of retinal hemodynamics in diabetic rats by increased expression and action of endothelin-1. Investigative Ophthalmology and Visual Science. 1996;**37**:2504-2518

[32] Dahl-Jorgensen K. Diabetic microangiopathy. Acta Paediatrica (Oslo, Norway: 1992) Supplement. 1998;**425**:31-34

[33] Blair NP, Feke GT, Morales-Stoppello J, Riva CE, Goger DG, Collas G, et al. Prolongation of the retinal mean circulation time in diabetes. Archives of Ophthalmology (Chicago, IL: 1960). 1982;**100**:764-768

[34] Cuypers MH, Kasanardjo JS, Polak BC. Retinal blood flow changes in diabetic retinopathy measured with the Heidelberg scanning laser Doppler flowmeter. Graefe's Archive for Clinical and Experimental Ophthalmology = Albrecht von Graefes Archiv fur klinische und experimentelle Ophthalmologie. 2000;**238**:935-941

[35] Goebel W, Lieb WE, Ho A, Sergott RC, Farhoumand R, Grehn F. Color Doppler imaging: A new technique to assess orbital blood flow in patients with diabetic retinopathy. Investigative Ophthalmology and Visual Science. 1995;**36**:864-870

[36] Pechauer AD, Hwang TS, Hagag AM, Liu L, Tan O, Zhang X, et al. Assessing total retinal blood flow in diabetic retinopathy using multiplane en face Doppler optical coherence tomography. Br J Ophthalmol. 2017 May 11. pii: bjophthalmol-2016-310042. DOI: 10.1136/bjophthalmol-2016-310042

[37] Grunwald JE, DuPont J, Riva CE. Retinal haemodynamics in patients with early diabetes mellitus. The British Journal of Ophthalmology. 1996;**80**:327-331

[38] Wang Y, Fawzi AA, Varma R, Sadun AA, Zhang X, Tan O, et al. Pilot study of optical coherence tomography measurement of retinal blood flow in retinal and optic nerve diseases. Investigative Ophthalmology and Visual Science. 2011;**52**:840-845

[39] PK Y, Balaratnasingam C, Cringle SJ, Mcallister IL, Provis J, Dao-Yi Y. Microstructure and network organization of the microvasculature in the human macula. Investigative Ophthalmology and Visual Science. 2010;**51**:6735-6743

[40] Campbell JP, Zhang M, Hwang TS, Bailey ST, Wilson DJ, Jia Y, et al. Detailed vascular anatomy of the human retina by projection-resolved optical coherence tomography angiography. Scientific Reports. 2017;**7**:42201

[41] Spaide RF, Klancnik JM, Cooney MJ. Retinal vascular layers imaged by fluorescein angiography and optical coherence tomography angiography. JAMA Ophthalmology. 2015;**133**:45-50

[42] de Carlo TE, Romano A, Waheed NK, Duker JS. A review of optical coherence tomography angiography (OCTA). International Journal of Retina and Vitreous. 2015;**1**:5

[43] Kwiterovich KA, Maguire MG, Murphy RP, Schachat AP, Bressler NM, Bressler SB, et al. Frequency of adverse systemic reactions after fluorescein angiography. Results of a prospective study. Ophthalmology. 1991;**98**(7):1139-1142

[44] Sim DA, Keane PA, Rajendram R, Karampelas M, Selvam S, Powner MB, et al. Patterns of peripheral retinal and central macula ischemia in diabetic retinopathy as evaluated by ultra-widefield fluorescein angiography. American Journal of Ophthalmology. 2014 Jul;**158**(1):144-153.e1. DOI: 10.1016/j.ajo.2014.03.009. Epub 2014 Apr 4

[45] Sim DA, Keane PA, Zarranz-Ventura J, Bunce CV, Fruttiger M, Patel PJ, et al. Predictive factors for the progression of diabetic macular ischemia. American Journal of Ophthalmology. 2013;**156**:684-92.e1

[46] Tam J, Martin JA, Roorda A. Noninvasive visualization and analysis of parafoveal capillaries in humans. Investigative Ophthalmology and Visual Science. 2010;**51**:1691-1698

[47] Hwang TS, Gao SS, Liu L, Lauer AK, Bailey ST, Flaxel CJ, et al. Automated quantification of capillary nonperfusion using optical coherence tomography angiography in diabetic retinopathy. JAMA Ophthalmology. 2016;**97239**:1

[48] Conrath J, Giorgi R, Raccah D, Ridings B. Foveal avascular zone in diabetic retinopathy: Quantitative vs qualitative assessment. Eye (London, England). 2005;**19**:322-326

[49] Lin AD, Lee AY, Zhang Q, Rezaei KA, Kinyoun J, Wang RK, et al. Association between OCT-based microangiography perfusion indices and diabetic retinopathy severity. Br

J Ophthalmol. 2017 Jul;**101**(7):960-964. DOI: 10.1136/bjophthalmol-2016-309514. Epub 2016 Nov 15

[50] Dimitrova G, Chihara E, Takahashi H, Amano H, Okazaki K. Quantitative retinal optical coherence tomography angiography in patients with diabetes without diabetic retinopathy. Investigative Ophthalmology and Visual Science. 2017;**58**:190-196

[51] Al-Sheikh M, Akil H, Pfau M, Sadda SR. Swept-source OCT angiography imaging of the Foveal avascular zone and macular capillary network density in diabetic retinopathy. Investigative Opthalmology and Visual Science. 2016;**57**:3907

[52] Ishibazawa A, Nagaoka T, Takahashi A, Omae T, Tani T, Sogawa K, et al. Optical coherence tomography angiography in diabetic retinopathy: A prospective pilot study. American Journal of Ophthalmology. 2015;**160**:35-44.e1

[53] Durbin MK, An L, Shemonski ND, Soares M, Santos T, Lopes M, et al. Quantification of retinal microvascular density in optical coherence tomographic angiography images in diabetic retinopathy. JAMA Ophthalmology. 2017;**135**:370-376

[54] Couturier A, Bonnin S, Erginay aLI, Massin P, Gaudric A, Tadayoni R. Capillary Plexus Anomalies in Diabetic Retinopathy on Optical Coherence Tomography. Retina. 2015 Nov;**35**(11):2384-91. DOI: 10.1097/IAE.0000000000000859

[55] Choi W, Waheed NK, Moult EM, Adhi M, Lee B, De Carlo T, Jayaraman V, Baumal CR, Duker JS, Fujimoto JG. Ultrahigh speed swept source optical coherence tomography angiography of retinal and choriocapillaris alterations in diabetic patients with and without retinopathy. Retina. 2017 Jan;**37**(1):11-21. DOI: 10.1097/IAE.0000000000001250

[56] Agemy Sa, Scripsema NK, Shah CM, Gentile RC, Hsiao Y-s, Zhou Q. Retinal Vascular Perfusion Density Mapping Using Optical Coherence Tomography Angiography in Normals and Diabetic Retinopathy Patients. Retina. 2015 Nov;**35**(11):2353-63. DOI: 10.1097/IAE.0000000000000862

[57] Salz Da, de Carlo TE, Adhi M, Moult E, Choi W, Baumal CR, et al. Select features of diabetic retinopathy on swept-source optical coherence tomographic angiography compared with fluorescein angiography and normal eyes. JAMA Ophthalmology. 2016:1-7

[58] Akihiro Ishibazawa TM, Shimizu K, Young-Seok Song AY. Evaluation of microaneurysms in diabetic retinopathy using different types of optical coherence tomography angiography. The Association for Research in Vision and Ophthalmology Conference, Baltimore. 2017. Poster A0091abstract

[59] Scarinci F, Nesper PL, Fawzi AA. Deep retinal capillary nonperfusion is associated with photoreceptor disruption in diabetic macular ischemia. American Journal of Ophthalmology. 2016;**168**:129-138

[60] Mauricio J, Barros BD, Leonardo D, Isaac C, Avila M. Diabetic retinopathy and OCT angiography : clinical findings and future perspectives. International Journal of Retina and Vitreous. Int J Retina Vitreous. 2017 Mar 13;**3**:14. DOI: 10.1186/s40942-017-0062-2. eCollection 2017

[61] Geirsdottir A, Palsson O, Hardarson SH, Olafsdottir OB, Kristjansdottir JV, Stefansson E. Retinal vessel oxygen saturation in healthy individuals. Investigative Ophthalmology and Visual Science. 2012;**53**:5433-5442

[62] Yip WF, Siantar R, Perera SA, Milastuti N, Ho KK, Tan B, et al. Reliability and determinants of retinal vessel oximetry measurements in healthy eyes. Investigative Ophthalmology and Visual Science. 2014;**55**:7104-7110

[63] Turksever C, Orgul S, Todorova MG. Reproducibility of retinal oximetry measurements in healthy and diseased retinas. Acta Ophthalmologica. 2015;**93**:e439-e445

[64] Palsson O, Geirsdottir A, Hardarson SH, Olafsdottir OB, Kristjansdottir JV, Stefánsson E. Retinal oximetry images must be standardized: A methodological analysis. Investigative Ophthalmology and Visual Science. 2012;**53**:1729-1733

[65] Jani P, Mwanza J-C, Billow K, Waters A, Moyer S, Garg S. Normative values and predictors of retinal oxygen saturation. Retina. 2014;**34**:394-401

[66] Akil H, Falavarjani K, Sadda S, Sadun A. Optical coherence tomography angiography of the optic disc: An overview. Journal of Ophthalmic and Vision Research. 2017;**12**:98

[67] Guduru A, Martz TG, Waters A, Kshirsagar AV, Garg S. Oxygen saturation of retinal vessels in all stages of diabetic retinopathy and correlation to ultra-wide field fluorescein angiography. Investigative Ophthalmology and Visual Science. 2016;**57**:5278-5284

[68] Khoobehi B, Firn K, Thompson H, Reinoso M, Beach J. Retinal arterial and venous oxygen saturation is altered in diabetic patients. Investigative Ophthalmology and Visual Science. 2013;**54**:7103-7106

[69] Hardarson SH, Stefansson E. Retinal oxygen saturation is altered in diabetic retinopathy. British Journal of Ophthalmology. 2012;**96**:560-563

[70] Jørgensen CM, Hardarson SH, Bek T. The oxygen saturation in retinal vessels from diabetic patients depends on the severity and type of vision-threatening retinopathy. Acta Ophthalmologica. 2014;**92**:34-39

[71] Hardarson SH. Retinal oximetry. Acta Ophthalmologica. 2013;**91**:1-47

[72] COGAN DG, KUWABARA T. Capillary shunts in the pathogenesis of diabetic retinopathy. Diabetes. 1963;**12**:293-300

[73] Ashton N. Vascular basement membrane changes in diabetic retinopathy. Montgomery lecture, 1973. The British Journal of Ophthalmology. 1974;**58**:344-366

[74] Holekamp NM, Shui Y-B, Beebe D. Lower intraocular oxygen tension in diabetic patients: Possible contribution to decreased incidence of nuclear sclerotic cataract. American Journal of Ophthalmology. 2006;**141**:1027-1032

[75] Jørgensen CM. Lack of differences in the regional variation of oxygen saturation in larger retinal vessels in diabetic maculopathy and proliferative diabetic retinopathy. British Journal of Ophthalmology. 2016. No pagination

[76] Stefansson E, Machemer R, de Juan EJ, McCuen BWn, Peterson J. Retinal oxygenation and laser treatment in patients with diabetic retinopathy. American Journal of Ophthalmology. 1992;**113**:36-38

[77] Jørgensen C, Bek T. Increasing oxygen saturation in larger retinal vessels after photocoagulation for diabetic retinopathy. Investigative Ophthalmology and Visual Science. 2014;**55**:5365-5369

[78] Torp TL, Kawasaki R, Wong TY, Peto T, Grauslund J. Changes in retinal venular oxygen saturation predict activity of proliferative diabetic retinopathy 3 months after panretinal photocoagulation. Br J Ophthalmol. 2017 Aug 1. pii: bjophthalmol-2017-310576. DOI: 10.1136/bjophthalmol-2017-310576

[79] Shimizu K, Kobayashi Y, Muraoka K. Midperipheral fundus involvement in diabetic retinopathy. Ophthalmology. 1981;**88**:601-612

[80] Niki T, Muraoka K, Shimizu K. Distribution of capillary nonperfusion in early-stage diabetic retinopathy. Ophthalmology. 1984;**91**:1431-1439

[81] Early Treatment Diabetic Retinopathy Study Research Group. Grading diabetic retinopathy from stereoscopic color fundus photographs – An extension of the modified Airlie House classification. ETDRS Report Number 10. Ophthalmology. 1991;**98**:786-806

[82] Early Treatment Diabetic Retinopathy Study Research Group. Treatment techniques and clinical guidelines for photocoagulation of diabetic macular edema. Early Treatment Diabetic Retinopathy Study Report Number 2. Ophthalmology. 1987;**94**:761-774

[83] Silva PS, Cavallerano JD, Sun JK, Soliman AZ, Aiello LM, Aiello LP. Peripheral lesions identified by mydriatic ultrawide field imaging: Distribution and potential impact on diabetic retinopathy severity. Ophthalmology. 2013;**120**:2587-2595

[84] Silva PS, Cavallerano JD, Haddad NMN, Kwak H, Dyer KH, Omar AF, et al. Peripheral lesions identified on ultrawide field imaging predict increased risk of diabetic retinopathy progression over 4 years. Ophthalmology. 2015;**122**:949-956

[85] Silva PS, Cavallerano JD, Tolls D, Omar A, Thakore K, Patel B, et al. Potential efficiency benefits of nonmydriatic ultrawide field retinal imaging in an ocular telehealth diabetic retinopathy program. Diabetes Care. 2014;**37**:50-55

[86] Price LD, Au S, Chong NV. Optomap ultrawide field imaging identifies additional retinal abnormalities in patients with diabetic retinopathy. Clinical Ophthalmology. 2015;**9**:527-531

[87] Silva PS, Cavallerano JD, Sun JK, Noble J, Aiello LM. Nonmydriatic ultrawide field retinal imaging compared with dilated standard 7-field 35-mm photography and retinal specialist examination for evaluation of diabetic retinopathy. Am J Ophthalmol. 2012 Sep;**154**(3):549-559.e2. DOI: 10.1016/j.ajo.2012.03.019. Epub 2012 May 23

[88] Silva PS, Cavallerano JD, Haddad NM, Tolls D, Thakore K, Patel B, et al. Comparison of nondiabetic retinal findings identified with nonmydriatic fundus photography vs ultrawide field imaging in an ocular telehealth program. JAMA Ophthalmology. 2016;**134**:330-334

[89] Purbrick RMJ, Izadi S, Gupta A, Victor Chong N. Comparison of optomap ultrawide-field imaging versus slit-lamp biomicroscopy for assessment of diabetic retinopathy in a real-life clinic. Clinical Ophthalmology. 2014;**8**:1413-1417

[90] Mackenzie PJ, Russell M, Ma PE, Isbister CM, Maberley DL. Sensitivity and specificity of the optos optomap for detecting peripheral retinal lesions. Retina (Philadelphia, PA). 2007;**27**:1119-1124

[91] Manjunath V, Papastavrou V, Steel DHW, Menon G, Taylor R, Peto T, et al. Wide-field imaging and OCT vs clinical evaluation of patients referred from diabetic retinopathy screening. Eye (London, England). 2015;**29**:416-423

[92] Nagiel A, Lalane RA, Sadda SR, Schwartz SD. Ultra-widefield fundus imaging: A review of clinical applications and future trends. Retina (Philadelphia, PA). 2016;**36**:660-678

[93] Wessel MM, Aaker GD, Parlitsis G, Cho M, D'Amico DJ, Kiss S. Ultra-wide-field angiography improves the detection and classification of diabetic retinopathy. Retina (Philadelphia, PA). 2012;**32**:785-791

[94] Silva PS, Dela Cruz AJ, Ledesma MG, van Hemert J, Radwan A, Cavallerano JD, et al. Diabetic retinopathy severity and peripheral lesions are associated with nonperfusion on Ultrawide field angiography. Ophthalmology 2015:1-8

[95] Sun JK, Aiello LP. The future of ultrawide field imaging for diabetic retinopathy pondering the retinal periphery. JAMA Ophthalmology. 2016;**134**:247-248

[96] Klein R, Klein BE, Moss SE, Davis MD, DeMets DL. The Wisconsin epidemiologic study of diabetic retinopathy. IV. Diabetic macular edema. Ophthalmology. 1984;**91**:1464-1474

[97] Grant MB, Afzal A, Spoerri P, Pan H, Shaw LC, Mames RN. The role of growth factors in the pathogenesis of diabetic retinopathy. Expert Opinion on Investigational Drugs. 2004;**13**:1275-1293

[98] Salam A, DaCosta J, Sivaprasad S. Anti-vascular endothelial growth factor agents for diabetic maculopathy. The British Journal of Ophthalmology. 2010;**94**:821-826

[99] Browning DJ, Glassman AR, Aiello LP, Beck RW, Brown DM, Fong DS, et al. Relationship between optical coherence tomography-measured central retinal thickness and visual acuity in diabetic macular edema. Ophthalmology. 2007;**114**:525-536

[100] Maheshwary AS, Oster SF, Yuson RMS, Cheng L, Mojana F, Freeman WR. The association between percent disruption of the photoreceptor inner segment-outer segment junction and visual acuity in diabetic macular edema. American Journal of Ophthalmology. 2010;**150**:63-7.e1

[101] Santos AR, Costa MÂ, Schwartz C, Alves D, Figueira J, Silva R, Cunha-Vaz JG. Optical coherence tomography baseline predictors for initial best-corrected visual acuity response to intravitreal anti-vascular endothelial growth factor treatment in eyes with diabetic macular edema: The chartres Study. Retina. 2017 May 2. DOI: 10.1097/IAE.0000000000001687

[102] Ito S-i, Miyamoto N, Ishida K, Kurimoto Y. Association between external limiting membrane status and visual acuity in diabetic macular oedema. The British Journal of Ophthalmology. 2013;**97**:228-232

[103] Sun JK, Lin MM, Lammer J, Prager S, Sarangi R, Silva PS, et al. Disorganization of the Retinal Inner Layers as a Predictor of Visual Acuity in Eyes With Center-Involved Diabetic Macular Edema. JAMA Ophthalmol. 2014 Nov;**132**(11):1309-16. DOI: 10.1001/jamaophthalmol.2014.2350

[104] Deak GG, Bolz M, Ritter M, Prager S, Benesch T, Schmidt-Erfurth U. A systematic correlation between morphology and functional alterations in diabetic macular edema. Investigative Ophthalmology and Visual Science. 2010;**51**:6710-6714

[105] Deak GG, Bolz M, Kriechbaum K, Prager S, Mylonas G, Scholda C, et al. Effect of retinal photocoagulation on intraretinal lipid exudates in diabetic macular edema documented by optical coherence tomography. Ophthalmology. 2010;**117**:773-779

[106] Bolz M, Schmidt-Erfurth U, Deak G, Mylonas G, Kriechbaum K, Scholda C. Optical coherence tomographic hyperreflective foci: A morphologic sign of lipid extravasation in diabetic macular edema. Ophthalmology. 2009;**116**:914-920

[107] Sophie R, Lu N, Campochiaro PA. Predictors of functional and anatomic outcomes in patients with diabetic macular edema treated with ranibizumab. Ophthalmology. 2015;**122**:1395-1401

[108] Gerendas BS, Prager S, Deak G, Simader C, Lammer J, Waldstein SM, et al. Predictive imaging biomarkers relevant for functional and anatomical outcomes during ranibizumab therapy of diabetic macular oedema. Br J Ophthalmol. 2017 Jul 19. pii: bjophthalmol-2017-310483. DOI: 10.1136/bjophthalmol-2017-310483

[109] Sun JK, Radwan SH, Soliman AZ, Lammer J, Lin MM, Prager SG, et al. Neural Retinal Disorganization as a Robust Marker of Visual Acuity in Current and Resolved Diabetic Macular Edema. Diabetes. 2015 Jul;**64**(7):2560-70. DOI: 10.2337/db14-0782. Epub 2015 Jan 29

[110] Radwan SH, Soliman AZ, Tokarev J, Zhang L, van Kuijk FJ, Koozekanani DD. Association of Disorganization of Retinal Inner Layers With Vision After Resolution of Center-Involved Diabetic Macular Edema. JAMA Ophthalmol. 2015 Jul;**133**(7):820-5. DOI: 10.1001/jamaophthalmol.2015.0972

[111] Sim DA, Keane PA, Zarranz-Ventura J, Fung S, Powner MB, Platteau E, et al. The effects of macular ischemia on visual acuity in diabetic retinopathy. Investigative Ophthalmology and Visual Science. 2013;**54**:2353-2360

[112] Nicholson L, Ramu J, Triantafyllopoulou I, Patrao NV, Comyn O, Hykin P, Sivaprasad S. Diagnostic accuracy of disorganization of the retinal inner layers in detecting macular capillary non-perfusion in diabetic retinopathy. Clin Exp Ophthalmol. 2015 Nov;**43**(8):735-41. DOI: 10.1111/ceo.12557. Epub 2015 Jun 24

[113] Gardner TW, Davila JR. The neurovascular unit and the pathophysiologic basis of diabetic retinopathy. Graefe's Archive for Clinical and Experimental Ophthalmology. Graefes Arch Clin Exp Ophthalmol. 2017 Jan;**255**(1):1-6. DOI: 10.1007/s00417-016-3548-y. Epub 2016 Nov 10

[114] Stem MS, Gardner TW. Neurodegeneration in the pathogenesis of diabetic retinopathy: Molecular mechanisms and therapeutic implications. Current Medicinal Chemistry. 2013;**20**:3241-3250

[115] Klaassen I, Van Noorden CJF, Schlingemann RO. Molecular basis of the inner blood-retinal barrier and its breakdown in diabetic macular edema and other pathological conditions. Progress in Retinal and Eye Research. 2013;**34**:19-48

[116] Cunha-vaz J, Ribeiro L, Lobo C. Progress in retinal and eye research phenotypes and biomarkers of diabetic retinopathy. Progress in Retinal and Eye Research. 2014;**41**:90-111

[117] del Zoppo GJ. The neurovascular unit in the setting of stroke. Journal of Internal Medicine. 2010;**267**:156-171

[118] Zlokovic BV. The blood-brain barrier in health and chronic neurodegenerative disorders. Neuron. 2008;**57**:178-201

[119] Drasdo N, Chiti Z, Owens DR, North RV. Effect of darkness on inner retinal hypoxia in diabetes. Lancet (London, England). 2002;**359**:2251-2253

[120] Gualtieri M, Bandeira M, Hamer RD, Damico FM, Moura ALA, Ventura DF. Contrast sensitivity mediated by inferred magno- and parvocellular pathways in type 2 diabetics with and without nonproliferative retinopathy. Investigative Ophthalmology and Visual Science. 2011;**52**:1151-1155

[121] Tzekov R, Arden GB. The electroretinogram in diabetic retinopathy. Survey of Ophthalmology. 1999;**44**:53-60

[122] Han Y, Bearse MAJ, Schneck ME, Barez S, Jacobsen CH, Adams AJ. Multifocal electroretinogram delays predict sites of subsequent diabetic retinopathy. Investigative Ophthalmology and Visual Science. 2004;**45**:948-954

[123] Harrison WW, Bearse MAJ, Ng JS, Jewell NP, Barez S, Burger D, et al. Multifocal electroretinograms predict onset of diabetic retinopathy in adult patients with diabetes. Investigative Ophthalmology and Visual Science. 2011;**52**:772-777

[124] Kern TS, Barber AJ. Retinal ganglion cells in diabetes. The Journal of Physiology. 2008;**586**:4401-4408

[125] Barber AJ. A new view of diabetic retinopathy: A neurodegenerative disease of the eye. Progress in Neuro-Psychopharmacology and Biological Psychiatry. 2003;**27**:283-290

[126] Chen Y, Li J, Yan Y, Shen X. Diabetic macular morphology changes may occur in the early stage of diabetes. BMC Ophthalmology. 2016;**16**:12

[127] van Dijk HW, Verbraak FD, Kok PHB, Garvin MK, Sonka M, Lee K, et al. Decreased retinal ganglion cell layer thickness in patients with type 1 diabetes. Investigative Ophthalmology and Visual Science. 2010;**51**:3660-3665

[128] Araszkiewicz A, Zozulińska-Ziółkiewicz D, Meller M, Bernardczyk-Meller J, Piłaciński S, Rogowicz-Frontczak A, et al. Neurodegeneration of the retina in type 1 diabetic patients. Polskie Archiwum Medycyny Wewnetrznej. 2012;**122**:464-470

[129] Sohn EH, van Dijk HW, Jiao C, Kok PHB, Jeong W, Demirkaya N, et al. Retinal neurodegeneration may precede microvascular changes characteristic of diabetic retinopathy in diabetes mellitus. Proc Natl Acad Sci U S A. 2016 May 10;**113**(19):E2655-64. DOI: 10.1073/pnas.1522014113. Epub 2016 Apr 25

[130] Verma A, Raman R, Vaitheeswaran K, Pal SS, Laxmi G, Gupta M, et al. Does neuronal damage precede vascular damage in subjects with type 2 diabetes mellitus and having no clinical diabetic retinopathy? Ophthalmic Research. 2011;**47**:202-207

[131] Zhu T, Ma J, Li Y, Zhang Z. Association between retinal neuronal degeneration and visual function impairment in type 2 diabetic patients without diabetic retinopathy. Science China Life Sciences. 2015;**58**:550-555

[132] Chhablani J, Sharma A, Goud A, Peguda HK, Rao HL, Begum VU, et al. Neurodegeneration in type 2 diabetes: Evidence from spectral-domain optical coherence tomography. Investigative Opthalmology and Visual Science. 2015;**56**:6333

[133] van Dijk HW, Verbraak FD, Stehouwer M, Kok PH, Garvin MK, Sonka M, DeVries JH, Schlingemann RO, Abràmoff MD. Association of visual function and ganglion cell layer thickness in patients with diabetes mellitus type 1 and no or minimal diabetic retinopathy. Vision Res. 2011 Jan 28;**51**(2):224-8. DOI: 10.1016/j.visres.2010.08.024. Epub 2010 Aug 27

[134] Frydkjaer-Olsen U, Soegaard Hansen R, Simó R, Cunha-Vaz J, Peto T, Grauslund J; EUROCONDOR. Correlation between Retinal Vessel Calibre and Neurodegeneration in Patients with Type 2 Diabetes Mellitus in the European Consortium for the Early Treatment of Diabetic Retinopathy (EUROCONDOR). Ophthalmic Res. 2016;**56**(1):10-6. DOI: 10.1159/000444396. Epub 2016 Apr 8

[135] Bearse MA, Adams AJ, Han Y, Schneck ME, Ng J, Bronson-Castain K, et al. A multifocal electroretinogram model predicting the development of diabetic retinopathy. Progress in Retinal and Eye Research. 2006;**25**:425-448

[136] Srinivasan S, Pritchard N, Sampson GP, Edwards K, Vagenas D, Russell AW, et al. Focal loss volume of ganglion cell complex in diabetic neuropathy. Clin Exp Optom. 2016 Nov;**99**(6):526-534. DOI: 10.1111/cxo.12379. Epub 2016 Mar 29

[137] Simó R, Sundstrom JM, Antonetti DA. Ocular anti-VEGF therapy for diabetic retinopathy: The role of VEGF in the pathogenesis of diabetic retinopathy. Diabetes Care. 2014;**37**:893-899

[138] Simó R, Hernández C; European Consortium for the Early Treatment of Diabetic Retinopathy (EUROCONDOR). Neurodegeneration in the diabetic eye: new insights and therapeutic perspectives. Trends Endocrinol Metab. 2014 Jan;**25**(1):23-33. DOI: 10.1016/j.tem.2013.09.005. Epub 2013 Nov 1

[139] Ma A-A, Fares U, Suleman H, Lowe J, Dua HS. Architecture and distribution of human corneal nerves. The British Journal of Ophthalmology. 2010;**94**:784-789

[140] Hertz P, Bril V, Orszag A, Ahmed A, Ng E, Nwe P, et al. Reproducibility of in vivo corneal confocal microscopy as a novel screening test for early diabetic sensorimotor polyneuropathy. Diabetic Medicine. 2011;**28**:1253-1260

[141] Ziegler D, Papanas N, Zhivov A, Allgeier S, Winter K, Ziegler I, et al. Early detection of nerve fiber loss by corneal confocal microscopy and skin biopsy in recently diagnosed type 2 diabetes. Diabetes. 2014;**63**:2454-2463

[142] Chen X, Graham J, Dabbah MA, Petropoulos IN, Ponirakis G, Asghar O, et al. Small nerve Fiber quantification in the diagnosis of diabetic sensorimotor polyneuropathy: Comparing corneal confocal microscopy with Intraepidermal nerve Fiber density. Diabetes Care. 2015;**6**:1138-1144

[143] The global burden of diabetic foot disease. Boulton AJ, Vileikyte L, Ragnarson-Tennvall G, Apelqvist J. Lancet. 2005 Nov 12;**366**(9498):1719-24

[144] Kaku M, Vinik A, Simpson DM. Pathways in the diagnosis and management of diabetic polyneuropathy. Current Diabetes Reports. 2015;**15**:1-16

[145] Petropoulos IN, Alam U, Fadavi H, Asghar O, Green P, Ponirakis G, et al. Corneal nerve loss detected with corneal confocal microscopy is symmetrical and related to the severity of diabetic polyneuropathy. Diabetes Care. 2013;**36**:3646-3651

[146] Nitoda E, Kallinikos P, Pallikaris A, Moschandrea J, Amoiridis G, Ganotakis ES, et al. Correlation of diabetic retinopathy and corneal neuropathy using confocal microscopy. Current Eye Research. 2012;**37**:898-906

[147] Bitirgen G, Ozkagnici A, Malik RA, Kerimoglu H. Corneal nerve fibre damage precedes diabetic retinopathy in patients with type 2 diabetes mellitus. Diabetic Medicine. 2014;**31**:431-438

[148] Zhivov A, Winter K, Hovakimyan M, Peschel S, Harder V, Schober H-C, et al. Imaging and quantification of subbasal nerve plexus in healthy volunteers and diabetic patients with or without retinopathy. PLoS One. 2013;**8**:e52157

[149] Messmer EM, Schmid-Tannwald C, Zapp D, Kampik A. Vivo confocal microscopy of corneal small fiber damage in diabetes mellitus. Graefe's archive for clinical and experimental ophthalmology = Albrecht von Graefes Archiv fur klinische und experimentelle Ophthalmologie. 2010;**248**:1307-1312

Chapter 3

Interphotoreceptor Retinoid-Binding Protein Implications in Diabetic Retinopathy

Kevin Bermea

Additional information is available at the end of the chapter

http://dx.doi.org/10.5772/intechopen.72835

Abstract

The interphotoreceptor retinoid-binding protein (IRBP) is the most abundant protein in the interphotoreceptor matrix (IPM) and its levels decrease beginning in the early stages of diabetes. IRBP participates in the delivery of retinoids between retinal cells to carry out the visual cycle and also protects those retinoids against degradation in the IPM. IRBP deficiency is related to several conditions such as retinitis pigmentosa, cone-rod dystrophy, increased oxidative stress in the photoreceptors, and myopia. Decreased IRBP levels in diabetes could be due to the secretion of inflammatory cytokines and a direct effect of hyperglycemia on the photoreceptors. It is known that prior to the occurrence of vascular changes in diabetic retina, electrophysiological alterations occur on early potentials. Alterations on the photoreceptor outer segments and increased oxidative stress indicate an important affliction of the photoreceptors from early stages. Due to the importance of IRBP in photoreceptor wellness, its decreased levels may be linked to early photoreceptor affection. More studies are required to describe in detail the whole impact that decreased levels of IRBP in diabetes may have.

Keywords: interphotoreceptor retinoid-binding protein, IRBP, visual cycle, oxidative stress, ER-stress, light damage, retinitis pigmentosa, cone-rod dystrophy, photoreceptor damage, photoreceptor, S-cones, M-cones, outer segment, diabetes, neurodegeneration

1. Introduction

Typically, the pathological changes described in diabetic retina involve neovascularization and increased blood vessel permeability, a condition known as diabetic retinopathy (DR). Early changes that occur prior to the vascular affection have been acquiring more interest by the scientific community. Retinal proteomic analysis, functional and histopathological studies have revealed alteration in the levels of some proteins and a neurodegeneration state mainly involving ganglion and photoreceptor cells accompanied by reactive gliosis [1–5].

The interphotoreceptor retinoid-binding protein (IRBP), which is the most abundant protein in the interphotoreceptor matrix (IPM) [6–10], is one of the principal elements altered in early stages of diabetes. This protein is expressed mainly by the cone and rod photoreceptor cells [11–13]. It binds to the retinoids in the interphotoreceptor matrix and facilitates their exchange between the IPM and the cells that carry out the visual cycle [14–16].

Aside from the retinoid delivery, IRBP protects retinoids against degradation [17], the retinal cells from oxidative stress and light-induced injury [18, 19], and is important for eye development [20].

2. Pathologies associated with IRBP deficiency

In pathological conditions in which a deficiency of IRBP exists, an important anomaly of the photoreceptor cells and the visual cycle can be detected which leads in some cases to the development of retinitis pigmentosa, accumulation of the cytotoxic bis-retinoid A2E, cone-rod photoreceptor dystrophy and an elongated myopic eye shape [20–25].

IRBP is linked to an autosomal recessive form of retinitis pigmentosa. A heterozygous T-C transition at the position 3024 [26] and a missense mutation of D1080N [22] have been identified. *In vitro* studies of this mutation have shown that it produces a non-secreted protein that induces endoplasmic reticular (ER) stress [27].

Other studies correlate the presence of *IRBP* gene mutations and the occurrence of high myopia in humans. This myopia was accompanied with retinal dystrophy observed by ocular coherence tomography (OCT) and electroretinography (ERG). The ERG showed a delay and reduction in the amplitude of the waves corresponding to the cone response. The *IRPB* gene mutations were c.3454G > T;p.E1152 and c.1530 T > A;p.Y510 which were predicted to lead to a nonsense mediated decay with a complete loss of IRBP function [21]. These findings correlate with animal studies in which IRBP−/− mice have shown ERG alterations and histological findings affecting cones [25]. This animal model has also shown alterations in eye shape and visual acuity [20].

The relationship between IRBP deficiency and accumulation of the lipofuscin precursor A2E has only be demonstrated experimentally on two different animal models. *IRBP−/−* mice have been shown by HPLC a retinal A2E increase of 2.7-fold [25]. Another study using an animal model with Müller cell dysfunction found a decreased expression of IRBP which was also accompanied with accumulation of A2E [24].

3. Diabetes and IRBP levels

Considering visual cycle components, decreased IRBP expression is one of the most characteristic changes in diabetes. Many studies have evaluated the changes in protein levels and IRBP expression and also attempted to explain the reasons for its depletion.

One study revealed decreased expression of IRBP determined by both qPCR and protein quantification on post-mortem samples of diabetic patients [28]. Another study showed that this decreased expression directly correlated with the evolution of the DR, and also tested the effect of glucose and inflammatory cytokines on IRBP expression *in vitro*. They found that high glucose, TNF-α and IL-1β were able to reduce IRBP's expression [29]. A recent study found decreased IRBP levels in diabetic rats and this finding was accompanied by decreased levels of 11-cRAL and rhodopsin synthesis [30].

The precise mechanisms responsible for the decreased IRBP levels remain unclear. It is known that high glucose and some circulating fatty acids can induce the secretion of inflammatory cytokines by Müller cells [31, 32]. Despite evidence that high levels of glucose and inflammatory cytokines are able to decrease the expression of IRBP [24, 29], other mechanisms may be involved. With the early onset of diabetes, photoreceptors undergo oxidative stress resulting in increased nitrosative-oxidative stress [33, 34]. This biochemical stress can induce damage to proteins promoting their degradation [35]. The unfolded protein response (UPR) has been detected to be active in photoreceptor cells in animal studies [36]; however no studies have linked this process to decreased IRBP levels.

Disruption of the external limiting membrane (ELM) and the outer retinal barrier (ORB) may play a role in leaking of IRBP into the outer nuclear layer or Bruch's membrane. Studies of animals in diabetic conditions have shown decreased occluding abilities in the Müller cell tight junctions compromising the external limiting membrane [37]. Also retinal pigment epithelium (RPE) dysfunction in early stage diabetes has been described in animal models [38]. It is still unclear the impact of these mechanisms over the IRBP levels.

4. Outcomes of IRBP's decreased levels in diabetes

Due to its importance on the visual cycle, it is expected that decreased levels of IRBP produce electrophysiological and morphological changes that manifest itself in the damage to the photoreceptors and the impaired visual cycle.

Deficit of blue-flicker discrimination has been observed in the early stages of diabetes [39]. ERGs have revealed lower oscillatory potential amplitudes suggesting alterations in the photoreceptors and the vision cycle [40–42]. Additionally, color vision has been shown to be altered in these early diabetes stages. Adaptometry studies have also shown alteration in diabetes; even with transient hyperglycemia a patient can have a delay in dark adaptation [43–45].

One study in *Meriones shawi*, an animal model with a human-like macula, after streptozotocin-induced diabetes showed alterations in the morphology of the photoreceptor outer segments. Interestingly, the foveal cones appear to be mostly affected revealing a loss of approximately 30% of the M-cones 7 weeks after type 2 diabetes was induced in the animals [46]. Studies in rats also have shown alterations in the photoreceptor outer segments with the S-cones and the M-cones most severely affected [47].

It has been found that glucose levels can influence the vision cycle rhodopsin regeneration ratio [48, 49]. Recently, one research group found depletion of rhodopsin regeneration with an accompanying decrease in STRA6, IRBP, and 11-cis retinal (11-cRAL) in a diabetic animal model [30].

5. Future directions

IRBP deficiency in diabetes could importantly impact DR progression although the relationship between its levels and the complications in diabetes remain unclear. Previous evidence suggest that it potentially impacts DR outcomes. In addition, some retinoid analogues have shown to be beneficial in the prevention of early stage DR due to their antioxidant properties [50, 51]. IRBP has been shown to have these anti-oxidant properties against some vision cycle retinoid sub-products [18].

IRBP deficiency can promote the accumulation of the cytotoxic bis-retinoid A2E. This molecule has been described to be involved in the pathogenesis of age-related macular degeneration (AMD) [52, 53] and Stargardt disease [54]. A2E is known to be able to produce cytotoxicity by destabilizing membranes, generating reactive oxygen species and producing photo-oxidation [55–58]. Since A2E is a lipofuscin precursor, fundus autofluorescence can be clinically used to detect its presence [59, 60]. However, hard exudates can decrease autofluorescence interfering with the evaluation of lipofuscin [61]. It would be expected that this accumulation of lipofuscin precursors in diabetes would increase the risk for developing AMD. Many studies have shown contradictory results and this relationship has not been established [62–65]. The actual accumulation, as well as the role of A2E in diabetes complications, is unclear and require further investigation.

It is important to reveal the mechanisms responsible for decreased IRBP in diabetes and to establish its role in DR in order to establish novel approaches for the prevention of these vision threatening events.

Author details

Kevin Bermea

*Address all correspondence to: kevchh89@hotmail.com

University of Texas Rio Grande Valley, Edinburg, Texas, USA

References

[1] Barber AJ, Lieth E, Khin SA, Antonetti DA, Buchanan AG, Gardner TW. Neural apoptosis in the retina during experimental and human diabetes. Early onset and effect of insulin. Journal of Clinical Investigation. 1998;**102**:783-791

[2] Tavares Ferreira J, Alves M, Dias-Santos A, Costa L, Santos BO, Cunha JP, Papoila AL, Abegão Pinto L. Retinal neurodegeneration in diabetic patients without diabetic retinopathy. Investigative Ophthalmology & Visual Science. 2016;**57**:6455-6460

[3] Carrasco E, Hernández C, de Torres I, Farrés J, Simó R. Lowered cortistatin expression is an early event in the human diabetic retina and is associated with apoptosis and glial activation. Molecular Vision. 2008;**14**:1496-1502

[4] Park SH, Park JW, Park SJ, Kim KY, Chung JW, Chun MH, Oh SJ. Apoptotic death of photoreceptors in the streptozotocin-induced diabetic rat retina. Diabetologia. 2003;**46**:1260-1268

[5] Lieth E, Barber AJ, Xu B, Dice C, Ratz MJ, Tanase D, Strother JM. Glial reactivity and impaired glutamate metabolism in short-term experimental diabetic retinopathy. Penn State Retina Research Group. Diabetes. 1998;**47**:815-820

[6] Carter-Dawson L, Burroughs M. Differential distribution of interphotoreceptor retinoid-binding protein (IRBP) around retinal rod and cone photoreceptors. Current Eye Research. 1989;**8**:1331-1334

[7] Anderson DH, Neitz J, Saari JC, Kaska DD, Fenwick J, Jacobs GH, Fisher SK. Retinoid-binding proteins in cone-dominant retinas. Investigative Ophthalmology & Visual Science. 1986;**27**:1015-1026

[8] Schneider BG, Papermaster DS, Liou GI, Fong SL, Bridges CD. Electron microscopic immunocytochemistry of interstitial retinol-binding protein in vertebrate retinas. Investigative Ophthalmology & Visual Science. 1986;**27**:679-688

[9] Gonzalez-Fernandez F, Landers RA, Glazebrook PA, Fong SL, Liou GI, Lam DMK, Bridges CDB. An extracellular retinol-binding glycoprotein in the rat eye—Characterization, localization and biosynthesis. Neurochemistry International. 1985;**7**:533-540

[10] Fong SL, Liou GI, Landers RA, Alvarez RA, Gonzalez-Fernandez F, Glazebrook PA, Lam DMK, Bridges CDB. Characterization, localization, and biosynthesis of an interstitial retinol-binding glycoprotein in the human eye. Journal of Neurochemistry. 1984;**42**:1667-1676

[11] Porrello K, Bhat SP, Bok D. Detection of interphotoreceptor retinoid binding protein (IRBP) mRNA in human and cone-dominant squirrel retinas by in situ hybridization. Journal of Histochemistry & Cytochemistry. 1991;**39**:171-176

[12] Hollyfield JG, Fliesler SJ, Rayborn ME, Fong SL, Landers RA, Bridges CD. Synthesis and secretion of interstitial retinol-binding protein by the human retina. Investigative Ophthalmology & Visual Science. 1985;**26**:58-67

[13] Gonzalez-Fernandez F, Landers RA, Glazebrook PA, Fong SL, Liou GI, Lam DM, Bridges CD. An extracellular retinol-binding glycoprotein in the eyes of mutant rats with retinal dystrophy: Development, localization, and biosynthesis. The Journal of Cell Biology. 1984;**99**:2092-2098

[14] Qtaishat NM, Wiggert B, Pepperberg DR. Interphotoreceptor retinoid-binding protein (IRBP) promotes the release of all-trans retinol from the isolated retina following rhodopsin bleaching illumination. Experimental Eye Research. 2005;**81**:455-463

[15] Betts-Obregon BS, Gonzalez-Fernandez F, Tsin AT. Interphotoreceptor retinoid-binding protein (IRBP) promotes retinol uptake and release by rat Müller cells (rMC-1) in vitro: Implications for the cone visual cycle. Investigative Ophthalmology & Visual Science. 2014;**55**:6265-6271

[16] Carlson A, Bok D. Promotion of the release of 11-cis-retinal from cultured retinal pigment epithelium by interphotoreceptor retinoid-binding protein. Biochemistry. 1992; **31**:9056-9062

[17] Gonzalez-Fernandez F, Betts-Obregon B, Yust B, Mimun J, Sung D, Sardar D, Tsin AT. Interphotoreceptor retinoid-binding protein protects retinoids from photodegradation. Photochemistry and Photobiology. 2015;**91**:371-378

[18] Lee M, Li S, Sato K, Jin M. Interphotoreceptor retinoid-binding protein mitigates cellular oxidative stress and mitochondrial dysfunction induced by all-trans-retinal. Investigative Ophthalmology & Visual Science. 2016;**57**:1553-1562

[19] Sun Z, Zhang M, Liu W, Tian J, Xu G. Photoreceptor IRBP prevents light induced injury. Frontiers in Bioscience (Landmark Ed). 2016;**21**:958-972

[20] Markand S, Baskin NL, Chakraborty R, Landis E, Wetzstein SA, Donaldson KJ, Priyadarshani P, Alderson SE, Sidhu CS, Boatright JH, Iuvone PM, Pardue MT, Nickerson JM.IRBP deficiency permits precocious ocular development and myopia. Molecular Vision. 2016;**22**:1291-1308

[21] Arno G, Hull S, Robson AG, Holder GE, Cheetham ME, Webster AR, Plagnol V, Moore AT. Lack of interphotoreceptor retinoid binding protein caused by homozygous mutation of RBP3 is associated with high myopia and retinal dystrophy. Investigative Ophthalmology & Visual Science. 2015;**56**:2358-2365

[22] den Hollander AI, McGee TL, Ziviello C, Banfi S, Dryja TP, Gonzalez-Fernandez F, Ghosh D, Berson EL. A homozygous missense mutation in the IRBP gene (RBP3) associated with autosomal recessive retinitis pigmentosa. Investigative Ophthalmology & Visual Science. 2009;**50**:1864-1872

[23] Wisard J, Faulkner A, Chrenek MA, Waxweiler T, Waxweiler W, Donmoyer C, Liou GI, Craft CM, Schmid GF, Boatright JH, Pardue MT, Nickerson JM. Exaggerated eye growth in IRBP-deficient mice in early development. Investigative Ophthalmology & Visual Science. 2011;**52**:5804-5811

[24] Zhu L, Shen W, Lyons B, Wang Y, Zhou F, Gillies MC. Dysregulation of inter-photoreceptor retinoid-binding protein (IRBP) after induced Müller cell disruption. Journal of Neurochemistry. 2015;**133**:909-918

[25] Jin M, Li S, Nusinowitz S, Lloyd M, Hu J, Radu RA, Bok D, Travis GH. The role of interphotoreceptor retinoid-binding protein on the translocation of visual retinoids and function of cone photoreceptors. The Journal of Neuroscience : The Official Journal of the Society for Neuroscience. 2009;**29**:1486-1495

[26] Valverde D, Vázquez-Gundín F, dR E, Calaf M, Fernández JL, Baiget M. Analysis of the IRBP gene as a cause of RP in 45 ARRP Spanish families. Autosomal recessive retinitis pigmentosa. Interstitial retinol binding protein. Spanish Multicentric and Multidisciplinary Group for Research into Retinitis Pigmentosa. Ophthalmic Genetics. 1998;**19**:197-202

[27] Li S, Yang Z, Hu J, Gordon WC, Bazan NG, Haas AL, Bok D, Jin M. Secretory defect and cytotoxicity: The potential disease mechanisms for the retinitis pigmentosa (rp)-associated interphotoreceptor retinoid-binding protein (IRBP). The Journal of Biological Chemistry. 2013;**288**:11395-11406

[28] García-Ramírez M, Canals F, Hernández C, Colomé N, Ferrer C, Carrasco E, García-Arumí J, Simó R. Proteomic analysis of human vitreous fluid by fluorescence-based difference gel electrophoresis (DIGE): A new strategy for identifying potential candidates in the pathogenesis of proliferative diabetic retinopathy. Diabetologia. 2007;**50**:1294-1303

[29] Garcia-Ramírez M, Hernández C, Villarroel M, Canals F, Alonso MA, Fortuny R, Masmiquel L, Navarro A, García-Arumí J, Simó R. Interphotoreceptor retinoid-binding protein (IRBP) is downregulated at early stages of diabetic retinopathy. Diabetologia. 2009;**52**:2633-2641

[30] Malechka VV, Moiseyev G, Takahashi Y, Shin Y, Ma J-X. Impaired rhodopsin generation in the rat model of diabetic retinopathy. The American Journal of Pathology. 2017;**187**:2222-2231

[31] Capozzi ME, McCollum GW, Cousins DB, Penn JS. Linoleic acid is a diabetes-relevant stimulator of retinal inflammation in human retinal Muller cells and microvascular endothelial cells. Journal of Diabetes & Metabolism. 2016;**7**:718

[32] Liu L, Zuo Z, Lu S, Liu A, Liu X. Naringin attenuates diabetic retinopathy by inhibiting inflammation, oxidative stress and NF-κB activation in vivo and in vitro. The Iranian Journal of Basic Medical Sciences. 2017;**20**:813-821

[33] Aboualizadeh E, Ranji M, Sorenson CM, Sepehr R, Sheibani N, Hirschmugl CJ. Retinal oxidative stress at the onset of diabetes determined by synchrotron FTIR widefield imaging: Towards diabetes pathogenesis. The Analyst. 2017;**142**:1061-1072

[34] Hernández-Ramírez E, Sánchez-Chávez G, Estrella-Salazar LA, Salceda R. Nitrosative stress in the rat retina at the onset of streptozotocin-induced diabetes. Cellular Physiology and Biochemistry. 2017;**42**:2353-2363

[35] Grune T, Reinheckel T, Joshi M. Davies KJ, Proteolysis in cultured liver epithelial cells during oxidative stress role of the multicatalytic proteinase complex, proteasome. The Journal of Biological Chemistry. 1995;**270**:2344-2351

[36] Shruthi K, Reddy SS, Reddy GB. Ubiquitin-proteasome system and ER stress in the retina of diabetic rats. Archives of Biochemistry and Biophysics. 2017;**627**:10-20

[37] Omri S, Omri B, Savoldelli M, Jonet L, Thillaye-Goldenberg B, Thuret G, Gain P, Jeanny JC, Crisanti P, Behar-Cohen F. The outer limiting membrane (OLM) revisited: Clinical implications. Clinical Ophthalmology (Auckland, N.Z.). 2010;**4**:183-195

[38] Samuels IS, Bell BA, Pereira A, Saxon J, Peachey NS. Early retinal pigment epithelium dysfunction is concomitant with hyperglycemia in mouse models of type 1 and type 2 diabetes. Journal of Neurophysiology. 2015;**113**:1085-1099

[39] Daley ML, Watzke RC, Riddle MC. Early loss of blue-sensitive color vision in patients with type I diabetes. Diabetes Care. 1987;**10**:777-781

[40] Bresnick GH, Palta M. Predicting progression to severe proliferative diabetic retinopathy. Archives of Ophthalmology. 1987;**105**:810-814

[41] Juen S, Kieselbach GF. Electrophysiological changes in juvenile diabetics without retinopathy. Archives of Ophthalmology. 1990;**108**:372-375

[42] Yamamoto S, Kamiyama M, Nitta K, Yamada T, Hayasaka S. Selective reduction of the S cone electroretinogram in diabetes. British Journal of Ophthalmology. 1996;**80**:973-975

[43] Greenstein V, Sarter B, Hood D, Noble K, Carr R. Hue discrimination and S cone pathway sensitivity in early diabetic retinopathy. Investigative Ophthalmology & Visual Science. 1990;**31**:1008-1014

[44] Tan NC, Yip WF, Kallakuri S, Sankari U, Koh YLE. Factors associated with impaired color vision without retinopathy amongst people with type 2 diabetes mellitus: A cross-sectional study. BMC Endocrine Disorders. 2017;**17**:29

[45] Holfort SK, Jackson GR, Larsen M. Dark adaptation during transient hyperglycemia in type 2 diabetes. Experimental Eye Research. 2010;**91**:710-714

[46] Hammoum I, Benlarbi M, Dellaa A, Szabó K, Dékány B, Csaba D, Almási Z, Hajdú RI, Azaiz R, Charfeddine R, Lukáts Á, Ben Chaouacha-Chekir R. Study of retinal neurodegeneration and maculopathy in diabetic Meriones shawi: A particular animal model with human-like macula. Journal of Comparative Neurology. 2017;**525**:2890-2914

[47] Énzsöly A, Szabó A, Kántor O, Dávid C, Szalay P, Szabó K, Szél Á, Németh J, Lukáts Á. Pathologic alterations of the outer retina in streptozotocin-induced diabetes. Investigative Ophthalmology & Visual Science. 2014;**55**:3686-3699

[48] Ostroy SE, Frede SM, Wagner EF, Gaitatzes CG, Janle EM. Decreased rhodopsin regeneration in diabetic mouse eyes. Investigative Ophthalmology & Visual Science. 1994;**35**: 3905-3909

[49] Ostroy SE, Friedmann AL, Gaitatzes CG. Extracellular glucose dependence of rhodopsin regeneration in the excised mouse eye. Experimental Eye Research. 1992;**55**:419-423

[50] Berkowitz BA, Kern TS, Bissig D, Patel P, Bhatia A, Kefalov VJ, Roberts R. Systemic retinaldehyde treatment corrects retinal oxidative stress, rod dysfunction, and impaired visual performance in diabetic mice. Investigative Ophthalmology & Visual Science. 2015; **56**:6294-6303

[51] Liu H, Tang J, Du Y, Lee CA, Golczak M, Muthusamy A, Antonetti DA, Veenstra AA, Amengual J, von Lintig J, Palczewski K, Kern TS. Retinylamine benefits early diabetic retinopathy in mice. The Journal of Biological Chemistry. 2015;**290**:21568-21579

[52] Ueda K, Zhao J, Kim HJ, Sparrow JR. Photodegradation of retinal bisretinoids in mouse models and implications for macular degeneration. Proceedings of the National Academy of Sciences of the United States of America. 2016;**113**:6904-6909

[53] Wu Y, Yanase E, Feng X, Siegel MM, Sparrow JR. Structural characterization of bisretinoid A2E photocleavage products and implications for age-related macular degeneration. Proceedings of the National Academy of Sciences of the United States of America. 2010; **107**:7275-7280

[54] Weng J, Mata NL, Azarian SM, Tzekov RT, Birch DG, Travis GH. Insights into the function of rim protein in photoreceptors and etiology of Stargardt's disease from the phenotype in abcr knockout mice. Cell. 1999;**98**:13-23

[55] Sparrow JR, Parish CA, Hashimoto M, Nakanishi K. A2E, a lipofuscin fluorophore, in human retinal pigmented epithelial cells in culture. Investigative Ophthalmology & Visual Science. 1999;**40**:2988-2995

[56] De S, Sakmar TP. Interaction of A2E with model membranes. Implications to the pathogenesis of age-related macular degeneration. The Journal of General Physiology. 2002; **120**:147-157

[57] Ben-Shabat S, Itagaki Y, Jockusch S, Sparrow JR, Turro NJ, Nakanishi K. Formation of a nonaoxirane from A2E, a lipofuscin fluorophore related to macular degeneration, and evidence of singlet oxygen involvement. Angewandte Chemie (International Ed. in English). 2002;**41**:814-817

[58] Rózanowska M, Jarvis-Evans J, Korytowski W, Boulton ME, Burke JM, Sarna T. Blue light-induced reactivity of retinal age pigment. In vitro generation of oxygen-reactive species. The Journal of Biological Chemistry. 1995;**270**:18825-18830

[59] Yung M, Klufas MA, Sarraf D. Clinical applications of fundus autofluorescence in retinal disease. International Journal of Retina and Vitreous. 2016;**2**:12

[60] Venkatesh P, Sagar P, Chawla R, Gogia V, Vohra R, Sharma YR. Evaluation of fundus autofluorescence patterns in age-related macular degeneration. International Journal of Ophthalmology. 2016;**9**:1779-1784

[61] Calvo-Maroto AM, Perez-Cambrodi RJ, Garcia-Lazaro S, Ferrer-Blasco T, Cerviño A. Ocular autofluorescence in diabetes mellitus. A review. Journal of Diabetes. 2016;**8**:619-628

[62] Leske MC, SY W, Hennis A, Nemesure B, Yang L, Hyman L, Schachat AP. Nine-year incidence of age-related macular degeneration in the Barbados Eye Studies. Ophthalmology. 2006;**113**:29-35

[63] Tan JS, Mitchell P, Smith W, Wang JJ. Cardiovascular risk factors and the long-term incidence of age-related macular degeneration: The Blue Mountains Eye Study. Ophthalmology. 2007;**114**:1143-1150

[64] Delcourt C, Michel F, Colvez A, Lacroux A, Delage M, Vernet MH. Associations of cardiovascular disease and its risk factors with age-related macular degeneration: The POLA study. Ophthalmic Epidemiology. 2001;**8**(4):237-249

[65] Fraser-Bell S, Wu J, Klein R, Azen SP, Hooper C, Foong AW, Varma R. Cardiovascular risk factors and age-related macular degeneration: The Los Angeles Latino Eye Study. American Journal of Ophthalmology. 2008;**145**:308-316

Chapter 4

Imaging of Hypoxia in Retinal Vascular Disease

Derrick J. Feenstra, Faye M. Drawnel and
Ashwath Jayagopal

Additional information is available at the end of the chapter

http://dx.doi.org/10.5772/intechopen.72252

Abstract

Retinal tissue hypoxia is a key mediator in the pathogenesis of many leading causes of irreversible vision loss, including diabetic retinopathy. Retinal hypoxia in diabetic retinopathy has been shown to drive the production of pro-inflammatory cytokines and pro-angiogenic growth factors. Together, these factors contribute to disease progression by causing unregulated growth of new blood vessels, increased vascular permeability and cell death within the retina. Studies have shown that retinal hypoxia precedes many of the pathologic events that occur during the progression of diabetic retinopathy such as angiopathy, microaneurysms, and capillary dropout. Therefore, early detection of hypoxia in the retinas of diabetic patients could help clinicians identify problems in patients before irreversible damage has occurred. Currently, oxygen sensitive electrodes remain the gold standard for direct measurement of oxygen tension within the retinal tissue; however the procedure is highly invasive and is therefore limited in its applicability towards preclinical models. Less invasive techniques such as retinal oximetry, phosphorescence-lifetime imaging, and hypoxia-sensitive fluorescent probes have shown promising diagnostic value in facilitating detection of oxygen imbalance correlated with neurovascular dysfunction in DR patients. This review highlights the current progress and potential of these minimally invasive hypoxia-imaging techniques in diabetic retinopathy.

Keywords: diabetic retinopathy, hypoxia, angiogenesis, neovascularization, imaging techniques

1. Introduction

1.1. Oxygen supply and consumption in the healthy retina

The retina is one of the most metabolically active sites of the entire body and is therefore dependent on a consistent supply of oxygen and other nutrients. In order to meet these metabolic demands, the retina requires two distinct blood supplies, the inner retinal circulation and choroidal circulation. The inner retinal circulation stems from the central retinal artery which enters the retina near the optic disc. From there, it branches to form the deep and superficial retinal capillary plexuses. In a healthy individual, these blood vessels are found only in the peripheral retina and do not enter into the avascular fovea. The central retinal artery is responsible for supplying the inner retina with oxygen and nutrients and receives about 20–30% of the blood flow to the retina [1]. The second blood supply is the choroidal circulation. The choroidal circulation is a dense network of capillaries located just posterior to the retinal pigment epithelium (RPE) cell layer and is responsible for supplying the outer retina (RPE and photoreceptors) with oxygen. Due to the high metabolic demand of the photoreceptors the choroid receives the majority (65–85%) of the blood that is supplied to the retina [1].

Studies in cats have used oxygen sensitive microelectrodes to measure oxygen tension (PO_2) in the various layers of the healthy retina. These studies have shown that oxygen levels are highest (≈60 mmHg) in the rod outer segment layer due to their close proximity to the oxygen saturated choroid (**Figure 1**) [2]. Oxygen tension drops to nearly 0 mmHg in the outer nuclear layer, indicating that the oxygen that is perfused from the choroidal circulation is consumed almost entirely by the photoreceptors during visual phototransduction [2]. Moving inward, PO_2 climbs gradually in the inner retina due to the inner retinal circulation, with two small spikes in PO_2 occurring in the deep (≈20 mmHg) and superficial (≈25 mmHg) retinal capillary plexuses [2]. Therefore, any vascular changes, especially in the inner retinal circulation can lead to tissue hypoxia since the choroidal circulation cannot adequately supply oxygen to the inner retina. Because of this, perturbations in oxygen supply play a significant role in many of the most common vision threating diseases including age-related macular degeneration (AMD) [3–6], glaucoma [7, 8], retinopathy of prematurity [9–11], and diabetic retinopathy (DR) [2, 12–15].

1.2. Hypoxia in diabetic retinopathy

Hypoxia has been implicated as a potential key contributor to the pathogenesis of many retinal diseases, including diabetic retinopathy (DR). The cellular hypoxia response is transcriptionally regulated by hypoxia inducible factors (HIFs) [16, 17], heterodimeric complexes comprising oxygen-sensing HIF1/2/3α subunits and HIFβ. The HIF alpha subunits share common features, although HIF3α has a distinct structure and is found in multiple variants which exert different transcriptional outcomes [18, 19]. Under normoxic conditions, proline residues in the oxygen-dependent degradation domain of HIFα are modified by oxygen-dependent prolyl hydroxylases (PHD) [20], creating a binding site for the von Hippel-Lindau (VHL) E3 ubiquitin ligase complex [21, 22]. HIFα bound by VHL is targeted for proteasomal destruction [23, 24], thus preventing transcriptional activity. However, during hypoxia HIFα proline hydroxylation is abrogated, stabilizing the protein. Transcriptional activity of HIF1α and HIF2α is also promoted during hypoxia, as hydroxylation of a key asparagine residue located in the transactivation domain is prevented, promoting interaction between HIF and the p300/ CBP transcriptional co-activator complex [25]. HIF3α, which lacks the key asparagine residue, is not subject to this regulatory mechanism [18]. The HIFα-HIFβ complex can activate transcription of genes with promoters featuring hypoxia response elements (HRE) including VEGF and erythropoietin (EPO).

http://dx.doi.org/10.5772/intechopen.72252

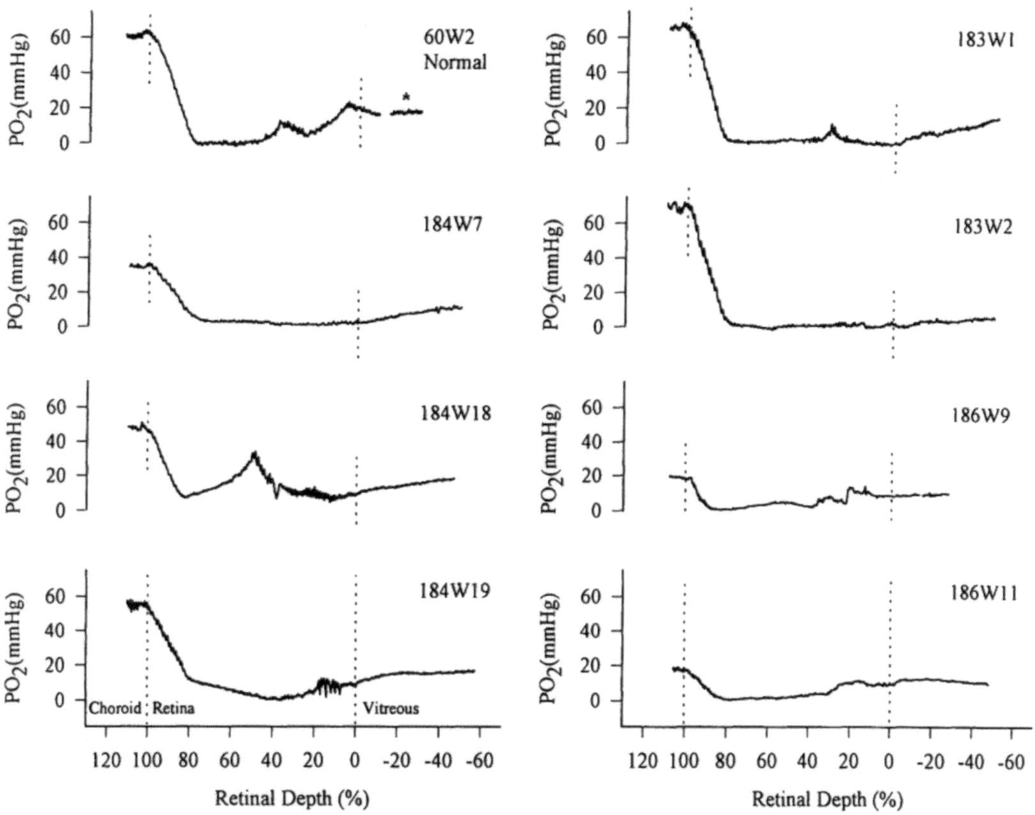

Figure 1. PO2 gradient across the retinal layers in a healthy (60 W2) and diabetic (all other tracings) cat. The tracing of the healthy cat shows normal oxygen perfusion in the choriocapillaris and inner retina. The diabetic cats show evidence of decreased oxygen perfusion in the inner retina and inadequate compensation by the choriocapillaris. Disclaimer: This figure has been reproduced with permission from original article by Linsenmeier et al. [2].

Although regulatory mechanisms are similar between HIF1α and HIF2α, expression of the proteins has been suggested to be confined to distinct cellular populations in the ischemic inner retina [26]. Expression of both HIF1α and HIF2α is temporally correlated with VEGF expression during retina ischemia [26, 27], and HIF2α haploinsufficiency has been shown to reduce pro-angiogenic factor expression and neovascularization in the oxygen-induced retinopathy (OIR) model [28]. Interestingly, PHD-dependent HIF1α degradation is also regulated by citric acid cycle intermediates such as succinate [29], which accumulate during hypoxia as oxygen tension is insufficient to support oxidative phosphorylation, leading to feedback inhibition of citric acid cycle enzymes [30]. Succinate inhibits PHD activity, further stabilizing HIF1α when cellular oxidative metabolism is compromised [29]. Succinate is also thought to have an addition role in the hypoxic retina, binding and signaling through the G protein coupled receptor 91 (GPR91) [31]. GPR91 regulates VEGF production in retinal ganglion cells via mitogen-activated protein kinase and prostaglandin signaling [32, 33] which contributes to the neovascular response following hypoxia [34].

Some of the hallmarks of DR progression which include the formation of acellular capillaries, capillary occlusion and associated nonperfusion could lead to this cellular hypoxia response in the diabetic retina [35–40]. Studies point toward an increase in the number of leukocytes and increased leukocyte adhesion as a source of capillary occlusion and tissue nonperfusion [36, 41, 42]. Furthermore, it has been shown that there is tissue hypoxia in the diabetic retina since the choriocapillaris cannot adequately provide the inner retina with oxygen. Linsenmeier et al. used oxygen-sensitive microelectrodes to directly measure PO_2 in the retinas of long term diabetic and non-diabetic cats (> 6 years) and showed that mean PO_2 was significantly lower in inner retina of diabetic (7.66 mmHg) compared to normal cats (16.42 mmHg) (**Figure 1**) [2]. These studies showed that hypoxia was evident early in disease progression, prior to observation of angiopathy, microaneurysms, hemorrhages and capillary dropout. Studies using magnetic resonance imaging (MRI) have also shown that there is a decrease in oxygen levels in galactosemic rats before retinal lesions appear [43]. These studies support the hypothesis that hypoxia may be a driving force in DR progression, rather than an outcome of other factors. Consistent with this hypothesis, hypoxia itself has been shown to stimulate production of a number of proangiogenic factors such as vascular endothelial growth factor (VEGF), one of the predominant targets of many therapeutic interventions in DR [44–48]. Steffanson et al. provided further evidence that oxygen delivery plays a crucial role in DR progression when they observed increased oxygen tension in the areas of the retina that had undergone panretinal photocoagulation compared to untreated areas [15]. This finding supports therapeutic strategies in DR which aim to restore normal oxygen supply in order to normalize disease.

Interestingly, although hypoxia has long been hypothesized as a potential driver of DR, it must be noted that there are a number of studies that were unable to detect the presence of hypoxia in the diabetic retina. Some studies in diabetic mice show that there is an initial decrease in retinal blood flow between three to 4 weeks due to arteriolar constriction, however arteriolar diameter and blood flow return to normal measurements at later time points of diabetes (12 weeks) [49–52]. Despite the initial decrease in blood flow these studies did not find any evidence of hypoxia in these animals at either 3 or 12 weeks of diabetes [53–55]. This may indeed be accounted for by compensatory vascular mechanisms in the rodent retina, such as autoregulation which may counteract early hypoxia in these species, and that onset of hypoxia may only occur at very late time points (>1.5 years) that are beyond typical published experimental endpoints in these models.

We are therefore in concurrence with a number of investigators in the ophthalmic and clinical research who identify retinal hypoxia as a significant mediator of initiation and progression of DR. Along with other researchers, we have sought to develop and translate strategies for optical detection of early retinal oxygen imbalance in patients to facilitate earlier clinical interventions and improved outcomes to reduce risk of future vision loss.

2. *In vivo* imaging of hypoxia in diabetic retinopathy

2.1. Overview of hypoxia sensing and imaging technologies

Oxygen-sensitive microelectrodes have long been considered the gold standard for measurement of PO_2 in tissues including the retina [2, 56–60]. While this technique gives an accurate and direct measurement of retinal tissue PO_2, there are many drawbacks, most importantly the highly invasive nature of the measurement, as it requires a direct puncture of the retinal tissue which prevents its use in clinics. Furthermore, oxygen imbalances in retinal vascular diseases such as DR originate largely from capillary occlusion and local changes in the retinal vasculature. These occlusions are likely to create small areas of regional hypoxia rather than an entirely hypoxic retinal tissue. Since oxygen sensitive microelectrodes provide point measurements that depend on the placement of the electrode this method will likely miss areas of focal hypoxia that are surrounded by large areas of normoxic tissue unless multiple measurements are made.

Other methods such as MRI have been used to provide insight into oxygen distribution within the retina and are less invasive than oxygen-sensitive microelectrodes. The advantages of MRI are that it is minimally invasive, offers a large field of view, and has no depth limitation. These MRI techniques are often based on the blood oxygenation level-dependent (BOLD) contrast that was first described by Ogawa et al. which rely on natural differences in MR signal between deoxygenated hemoglobin versus oxygenated hemoglobin [61–63], but can also utilize exogenous contrast agents for increased sensitivity as seen in Dynamic Contrast-Enhanced MRI (DCE-MRI) [64]. The use of MRI to detect changes in oxygen levels was first used in the brain but has since been adapted to visualize oxygen fluctuations in the diabetic retina. Berkowitz et al. have used MRI to show increases in blood retinal barrier permeability in rats after 8 months of diabetes [64] and changes in retinal oxygenation in galactosemia-induced diabetic-like retinopathy [43]. The primary limitation of MRI is that the information is typically displayed as either a cross section of the eye or single slice heat maps which are then pieced together to give an overview of the retina [43, 64–67]. This severely limits the techniques ability to provide the adequate resolution required to identify small regions of focal hypoxia in the diabetic retina.

Laser Doppler is another method that has been established to determine blood flow within the retinal vasculature but does not provide information on oxygen PO_2 within the retinal vasculature or tissue [68–70]. More recently however, a number of minimally invasive techniques have been established and adapted to measure oxygen tension optically and identify areas of regional hypoxia in the retina. These techniques take full advantage of the unique anatomy of the eye, which unlike other organs is readily accessible and easy to image due to the naturally transparent front of the eye. Methods such as dual wavelength and full spectral retinal oximetry, and also phosphorescence lifetime imaging all provide information on oxygen levels in the retinal vasculature. Other techniques such as hypoxia sensitive fluorescent probes can help to image hypoxic regions within the retinal tissue itself. These techniques are prime candidates for use in a clinical setting due to their minimally invasive nature and their ability to detect areas of focal hypoxia in the diseased retina.

This review will examine the advantages and disadvantages of the imaging techniques that have emerged as potential diagnostic tools for early detection of DR.

2.2. Dual wavelength retinal oximetry

Retinal oximetry is a non-invasive technique used to measure the percent of hemoglobin oxygen saturation (SO_2) in the retinal vasculature. Oximetry is based on the principle that oxygenated (HbO_2) and deoxygenated hemoglobin (Hb) have a different light absorption spectra. The use of spectrophotometric measurements to determine oxygen levels in large retinal vessels was first described by Hickam et al. in 1963, however their method required an independent arteriolar SO_2 measurement for external calibration [71]. Since this initial work, Delori [72], Beach [73], and Hardason et al. [74] have expanded the field by developing new techniques that decrease the invasiveness of retinal oximetry by eliminating the need for an external calibration measurement, while at the same time increasing sensitivity, accuracy, and reproducibility. More recently investigators have advanced this technology to develop new systems such as the Flow Oximetry System (FOS) that are able to measure oxygen saturation and blood flow within the retinal vasculature [75, 76].

Most studies have measured SO_2 by using dual wavelength oximetry. Here, two images at distinct wavelengths are taken simultaneously. A traditional fundus camera is attached to a beam splitter and digital camera in order to obtain digital images at multiple distinct wavelengths. One image is taken at an isobestic wavelength that is insensitive to differences in hemoglobin oxygen saturation. This is required for compensation against variables such as hematocrit, path length and light intensity that will not differ between the two images. In the image obtained from the isobestic wavelength there is no visual difference between oxygen saturated arteries compared to oxygen depleted veins. Simultaneously, a second image is taken at a wavelength that is sensitive to hemoglobin oxygenation. In this image there are clear differences between the oxygen saturated arteries and oxygen depleted veins. Software has now been developed to automatically detect blood vessels in order to help minimize other factors that contribute to optical density. This has led to highly reproducible measurements of SO_2 in large retinal vessels that can be depicted numerically or as a color map on the fundus image [74].

Since diabetes has been linked to abnormal oxygen distribution in the diabetic retina, retinal oximetry serves as a useful tool to examine changes in oxygen saturation in the retinal vasculature of diabetic patients. A number of studies have measured changes in venous (S_vO_2) and arterial (S_aO_2) oxygen saturation in patients with mild, moderate, or severe non-proliferative DR, and also proliferative DR. These studies consistently report increased S_vO_2 values as the severity of DR increases [77–83]. Interestingly, the results on whether arterial oxygen saturation changes during DR progression differ between studies. A number of studies have found that S_aO_2 increases with increased disease severity and these changes may not be present until the patient develops proliferative diabetic retinopathy [78–83], while others saw no difference in arterial oxygen saturation between DR patients in any stage compared to healthy individuals [77]. Studies using FOS saw no significant difference in either S_aO_2 or S_vO_2 between healthy individuals and DR patients, however identified significant changes in arteriovenous difference [75]. Together, these data indicate that there is increased venous oxygen saturation in DR patients; however due to the conflicting reports on S_aO_2 levels in DR patients, the cause of this S_vO_2 increase remains to be confirmed. This increase in venous oxygen saturation could be a result of decreased oxygen perfusion into the tissue which could lead to tissue hypoxia, but could also be a result of increased arterial oxygen saturation as observed in some reports, which could lead to subsequent increases in venous oxygen saturation with the same level of perfusion.

The advantages of retinal oximetry are that it is a non-invasive procedure that easily be performed in patients. This technique gives accurate and reliable measurements of SO_2 in the retinal vasculature to help provide insight into the dynamics of oxygen perfusion and consumption in these patients. Furthermore, retinal oximetry has shown that laser photocoagulation helps to improve oxygen delivery to the retina, and has therefore proven to be a useful tool in identifying the mechanisms of current DR treatments [15]. Another advantage of retinal oximetry is that systems are commercially available. However, since the use of retinal oximetry is restricted to the large retinal vessels, this technique might not adequately detect many of the changes seen in DR progression such as microaneurysms and acellular capillaries that occur in the small capillary beds of the retinal microvasculature. Furthermore, retinal oximetry provides a measurement of SO_2 levels within the vasculature, but does not give a direct measurement of what is happening within the retinal tissue itself. Whether the changes in vascular SO_2 observed in diabetic patients actually correlates to regions of hypoxia within the retina itself cannot be confirmed with retinal oximetry alone. This has been shown in studies examining the correlation between regional differences in oxygen saturation versus lesion formation in patients with proliferative diabetic retinopathy and diabetic maculopathy [84]. The study found that total SO_2 was increased in diabetic patients compared to healthy individuals indicating that there was decreased oxygen perfusion from the retinal vasculature, however the regional differences in SO_2 in the large retinal vessels did not correlate with the areas of retinal lesions [84]. This implies that other factors such as local changes in the microcirculation and within the tissue itself play a significant role in lesion formation and DR progression.

2.3. Full spectral imaging

In addition to dual wavelength oximetry, full spectral methods have also taken advantage of the differences between Hb and HbO_2 absorption spectra. Here, rather than using distinct isobestic and non-isobestic wavelengths to measure SO_2, a continuous range of wavelengths between visible and near-infrared spectrum are transmitted for measurement. Schweitzer et al. first described the technique by illuminating the retina with a narrow slit (1.5 × 40 mm) of light and capturing the image using an imaging ophthalmospectrometer, which consisted of a fundus camera adapted with a spectrograph coupled to an intensified CCD camera for detection [85, 86]. This allowed for collection of the full spectral data in a narrow band in a single dimension. Since then, full spectral imaging has developed into hyperspectral imaging (HSI) with algorithms used to construct a two dimensional image in order to visualize the data as an oxygen map [87–89]. Whereas this process originally took several seconds due to sequential acquisition of many single-dimension images, new technology allows for enough images to be taken to cover a 15 degree field with good spatial resolution in only a few milliseconds [90]. Today, HSI has been further developed into hyperspectral computed tomographic imaging spectroscopy (HCTIS), which in addition to giving detailed oxygen saturation maps, can give information about changes in the retina such as lesions, perfusion, and pigment density [90, 91].

Full spectral imaging has been used to examine oxygen imbalances in a number of vascular diseases including age-related macular degeneration [85], arteriovenous occlusion [88], and glaucoma [87, 89]. A limited number of studies have utilized full spectral imaging to examine changes in oxygen saturation in diabetic retinopathy. Kashani et al. used HCTIS to examine changes in S_aO_2 and S_vO_2 between healthy individuals and patients with DR and determined that S_aO_2 was significantly lower, while S_vO_2 was significantly higher in patients with proliferative DR [91]. This was confirmed by a significant difference in the arteriovenous difference between the two groups [91].

2.4. Phosphorescence-lifetime imaging

Phosphorescence-lifetime imaging is another minimally invasive technique that can be used to image PO_2 within the retina. The use of oxygen-dependent quenching of phosphorescence as a method of optical measurement of O_2 concentration was first described by Vanderkooi et al. [92, 93]. At the time, a similar method using oxygen-dependent quenching of fluorescence, rather than phosphorescence, had already been established [94]. The use of fluorescence however, was limited by low sensitivity to oxygen and by the fact that the decay in fluorescence brightness is rapid, which meant that only fluorescence intensity and not lifetime could be measured. Intensity measurements are complicated by variables such as solution composition and absorption in the tissue. By using phosphorescence, Vanderkooi et al. were able to measure lifetime, rather than intensity, due to the much slower decay in brightness of phosphorescence compared to fluorescence [92, 93]. It was observed that phosphorescence-lifetimes were directly dependent on oxygen concentration, with an increase in phosphorescence signal as PO_2 decreased, as described by a Stern-Volmer relationship [92, 93]. This technique was modified for use *in vivo* to measure PO_2 in the retinal and choroidal vasculature of large animals such as cats and pigs [95–97], and later for smaller animals such as mice and rats [98–104]. More recently Shahidi et al. have made significant advances by using phosphorescence-lifetime to image oxygen tension within the retinal tissue itself [105, 106]. This minimally invasive technique requires an intravenous injection of a phosphor that can be imaged using an intensified CCD camera to provide a clear image of retinal arteries, veins and even some capillaries with good spatial resolution.

To date, many of the studies utilizing phosphorescence-lifetime have sought to establish the technique and examine changes in oxygen tension during normal physiologic processes such as retinal response to light stimulation [68, 104]. A limited number of studies have utilized phosphorescence-lifetime to study oxygen imbalances in ischemic retinal diseases. Studies in a mouse model of oxygen-induced retinopathy (OIR) have shown that although there was no significant difference in arterial or venous PO2 between control and OIR mice, the arteriovenous difference was significantly higher in OIR mice [107]. This was attributed to a decreased vascular network in these OIR mice resulting in greater oxygen extraction from the larger vessels [107]. Other investigators have examined whether phosphorescence-lifetime imaging can be used to detect regions of local hypoxia created by laser photocoagulation. In these studies, a laser was used to create small (75 μm) focal lesions within the capillary network of the mouse retina [100]. Upon imaging and analysis using an oxygen map of the laser burn and surrounding area they observed a circular lesion with a central area of hypoxia (< 7 mmHg) that extended approximately 150–200 μm outward from the initial laser injury [100]. After imaging the lesion again 1 hour later there was no evidence of leakage of the phosphor into the tissue [100]. This study indicates that phosphorescence-lifetime imaging is a useful tool for identifying focal areas of regional hypoxia. Further experiments are needed to confirm whether these results translate into animal models of diabetic retinopathy.

The primary advantage of phosphorescence-lifetime imaging is that it is minimally invasive, requiring only an intravenous injection of a phosphor. These phosphors are readily available as nontoxic, water soluble forms so they can be easily dissolved in blood, providing further potential for use in a clinic. Furthermore, studies have shown that this technique is capable of identifying small areas of regional hypoxia created by focal lesions similar to those seen in DR [100]. This can be combined with traditional fundus photographs and fluorescein angiography to determine whether the areas of regional hypoxia correlate with the location of retinal lesions or leakage during the progression of DR. Finally, the information gathered can be displayed as an easy to read oxygen map showing retinal vascular function. The disadvantage of phosphorescence-lifetime imaging is similar to retinal oximetry in that it is a measurement of oxygen levels within the retinal vasculature rather than the retinal tissue itself. It must be noted however, that a number of studies have compared PO_2 measurements between the vasculature (using phosphorescence-lifetime) and a variety of tissues including the retina (using O_2 micro-electrodes) and found comparable results, with only slight decreases in PO2 within the tissue [95, 108]. The second disadvantage to phosphorescence-lifetime imaging is primarily due to the lack of evidence in animal models of DR. Although it has been proven useful in a number of vascular ischemic diseases that share commonalities with DR it would be necessary to confirm the applicability of phosphorescence-lifetime imaging in animal models of DR before proposing the technique as a potentially useful tool for determining PO_2 levels in DR patients.

2.5. Hypoxia-sensitive fluorescent probes

Another technique for imaging oxygen imbalances in the diabetic retina is the use of hypoxia-sensitive fluorescent probes. Hypoxia-sensitive compounds such as 2-nitroimidazoles are bioreduced by nitroreductases in hypoxic tissues (PO_2 < 10 mmHg) which leads to the formation of adducts with thiol containing proteins [109–113]. These compounds were originally discovered and used for detecting hypoxic areas within tumors and were imaged by autoradiography [112, 114]. Shortly after, immunohistochemical analysis was made possible by the production of antibodies that recognized the adducts formed by the reduced 2-nitroimidazoles and showed that the fluorescence intensity correlated with the severity of hypoxia [110, 111, 115]. More recently, 2-nitroimidazoles, such as pimonidazole, have been used to detect areas of hypoxia in a number of retinal vascular diseases, including extensive studies in diabetic retinopathy. *Ex-vivo* studies in non-diabetic and diabetic mice and rats have found significantly increased pimonidazole labeling in the retinas of even short-term diabetic mice and rats compared to their non-diabetic counterparts [53, 116–119]. Furthermore, the pimonidazole labeling was confirmed by increased staining of hypoxia inducible factor-1α (HIF-1α) and decreased ganglion cell function measured by electroretinogram (ERG) [53, 116].

Work by our group has sought to develop clinically useful hypoxia sensitive imaging agents by conjugating FDA-approved fluorescein dyes to adduct forming 2-nitroimidazoles. In preliminary studies, fluorescein isothiocyanate (FITC) was conjugated to a 2-nitroimidazole containing reagent to create the HYPOX-1 probe, and also to pimonidazole to create HYPOX-2. Both HYPOX-1 and HYPOX-2 formed adducts leading to accumulation in a variety of hypoxic retinal cells and allowed for imaging with excellent signal-to-noise ratio *in vitro* [120]. Furthermore, these imaging agents were capable of detecting hypoxic areas *ex vivo* in the retinas oxygen induced retinopathy (OIR) mice with no apparent toxicity [120]. Following the success of these fluorescent imaging agents, a new probe, HYPOX-3, was developed in order to create an "on-off" imaging agent for hypoxia [121]. Here, a near-infrared (NIR) imaging agent was coupled to Black Hole Quencher 3 (BHQ3), which had been shown to quench NIR dyes by Förster resonance energy transfer (FRET) [122]. Interestingly, BHQ3 features a hypoxia-sensitive azo-bond that is cleavable by azoreductases under hypoxic conditions [122, 123]. HYPOX-3 displayed high sensitivity and specificity in forming adducts in a variety of hypoxic retinal cells *in vitro* with no detectable toxicity [121]. The ability to detect hypoxia in retinal vascular disease animal models was examined using a laser-induced choroidal neovascularization (LCNV) mouse model. In RPE-choroid flatmounts, HYPOX-3 clearly identified hypoxic regions in LCNV mice and showed increased fluorescence around the lesion, with minimal fluorescence in control animals [121].

Due to the pharmacokinetics of HYPOX-1, -2, and -3, a new probe was designed with goal of creating an imaging agent for use *in vivo* with a potential for clinical application. This new probe, HYPOX-4, was characterized for *in vitro* and *in vivo* use and compared to immunostaining of pimonidazole-adducts [124, 125]. *In vitro,* HYPOX-4 displayed increasing fluorescence with decreasing oxygen concentration in a variety of different retinal cell lines [124]. *Ex vivo,* HYPOX-4 successfully identified avascular regions in the retinal flatmounts of OIR mice [124] (**Figure 2**) and hypoxic regions downstream of the occluded vein in the retinas of laser-induced retinal vein occluded (RVO) mice [125] (**Figure 3**). Using a micron IV imaging system, HYPOX-4 was then used for *in vivo* imaging of hypoxia in both the OIR and RVO mice. In both models, HYPOX-4 clearly identified areas of hypoxia *in vivo* [124, 125]. HYPOX-4 had no effect on proliferation (as measured by BrdU assay), toxicity (TUNEL), or function (ERG) [124].

The advantages to these hypoxia sensitive fluorescent probes are that they can be conjugated to already FDA approved fluorescent dyes and they allow for direct imaging of hypoxia within the retinal tissue, rather than the microvasculature. Furthermore, studies in the OIR mice have shown they are capable of detecting hypoxia in diseases where there is oxygen imbalance in the entire retina, while the RVO model has shown that they are also capable of detecting regional, focal hypoxia downstream of either a single or double vein occlusion. This alone makes these probes particularly useful in diseases such as DR where there is likely capillary occlusion leading to localized hypoxia within the retinal tissue. A disadvantage of these hypoxia sensitive fluorescent probes are that they only give an image of hypoxic areas without providing actual values for PO_2, although the PO_2 threshold for bioreduction and adduct formation is well characterized. Furthermore, these probes have been used in OIR and LCNV models to show their ability to identify focal hypoxia; however their use in models of diabetic retinopathy needs to be examined.

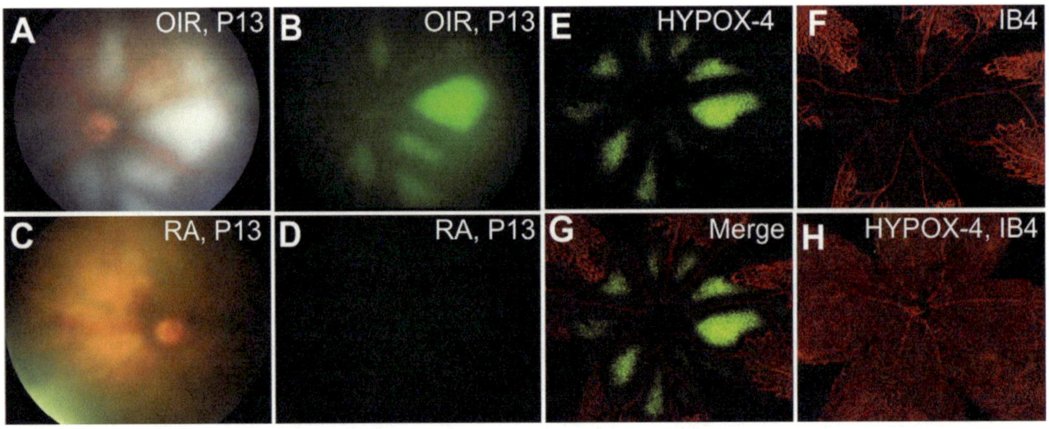

Figure 2. Imaging of HYPOX-4 in a mouse model of oxygen-induced retinopathy (OIR). Fundus and fluorescein channel *in vivo* images in OIR mice at P13 indicate accumulation of imaging probe in central, avascular hypoxic regions (A, B), which was not reflected by imaging in room air-reared age-matched controls (C, D). Findings in the OIR model correlated with microscopic imaging of retinal flatmounts (E, F, merged in G). Likewise, *ex vivo* analysis of room air control retinal flatmounts confirmed lack of HYPOX-4 accumulation in healthy, fully vascularized retinas (H). Disclaimer: This figure has been adapted from the original article by Uddin et al. [124] under Creative Commons Attribution 4.0 International License.

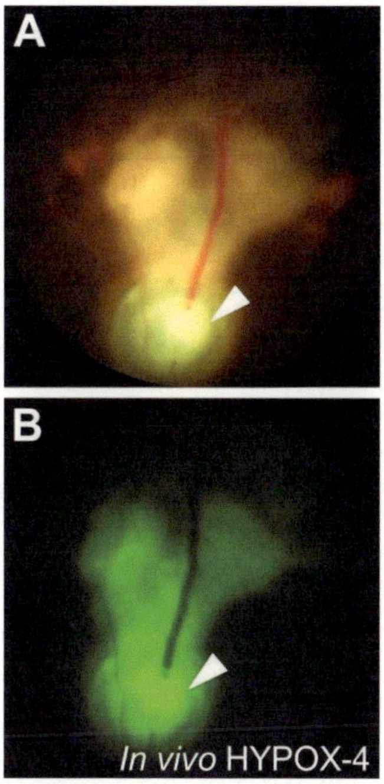

Figure 3. HYPOX-4 mediated retinal imaging of laser-induced retinal vein occlusion (RVO) in the mouse. HYPOX-4 injected 2 hours post vein occlusion with an argon photocoagulator in tandem with rose Bengal photosensitization. The imaging agent accumulated within the venous occlusion site (A, arrowhead) and downstream capillary bed (B). Disclaimer: this figure has been adapted from the original article by Uddin et al. [125] under Creative Commons Attribution 4.0 International License.

3. Summary

Hypoxia has been shown to play a significant role in DR progression. Hypoxia stimulates the production of a number of different pro-inflammatory cytokines (IL-1beta, TNF-a, ICAM-1) [7, 126, 127] and growth factors (VEGF and PDGF) [45, 47, 128, 129]that lead to neovascularization, increased vascular permeability and cell death. Studies have found that treatments such as laser photocoagulation provide benefits by restoring oxygen tension in the diabetic retina [15]. Furthermore, studies have indicated that oxygen imbalance actually precedes many of the pathological events that occur throughout the progression of diabetic retinopathy [2, 43, 130]. Therefore, early detection of hypoxic regions in the diabetic retina can potentially help clinicians choose appropriate treatment strategies before irreversible damage has already occurred.

New advances in imaging strategies allow for optical measurement the of oxygen levels *in vivo*. Oxygen sensitive microelectrodes have been the gold standard for direct measurement of oxygen levels in the retinal tissue, however the measurement is highly invasive and unable to consistently identify small areas of focal hypoxia. Together these factors prevent oxygen sensitive microelectrodes from being used in DR patients. More recently, less invasive techniques such as retinal oximetry, phosphorescence-lifetime imaging and hypoxia sensitive fluorescent probes have been developed in an effort to detect oxygen imbalances and allow for optical identification of hypoxic regions *in vivo*. Retinal oximetry and phosphorescence-lifetime have been used primarily to measure oxygen saturation in the retinal vasculature. These methods have been used in a number of different animal models and have shown that they can successfully identify regions of focal hypoxia surrounded by predominantly normoxic tissue, similar to what is hypothesized in DR. Hypoxia sensitive fluorescent probes differ from these techniques in that they detect hypoxic regions within the retina itself, rather than the microvasculature. These probes have been developed by the conjugation of fluorescein dyes, such as FITC, to 2-nitroimidazoles. These 2-nitroimidazoles are bioreduced by nitroreductases in under hypoxic conditions, causing them to aggregate within the hypoxic cells. A number of these hypoxia sensitive fluorescent probes have been developed and characterized for *in vitro, ex vivo,* and *in vivo* use with low toxicity.

The imaging techniques reviewed here have all been shown to optically identify regions of focal hypoxia *in vivo.* Clinically, these techniques can help to give an accurate depiction of oxygen imbalances within the diabetic retina before retinal pathologies are detectable and may therefore guide future treatment strategies in DR patients.

Author details

Derrick J. Feenstra, Faye M. Drawnel and Ashwath Jayagopal*

*Address all correspondence to: ash.jayagopal@gmail.com

Pharma Research and Early Development, Roche Innovation Center Basel, F. Hoffmann-La Roche, Ltd., Basel, Switzerland

References

[1] Kolb H. Simple anatomy of the retina. In: Kolb H, Fernandez E, Nelson R, editors. Webvision Organ. Retina Vis. Syst. Salt Lake City (UT): University of Utah Health Sciences Center; 1995

[2] Linsenmeier RA, Braun RD, McRipley MA, Padnick LB, Ahmed J, Hatchell DL, McLeod DS, Lutty GA. Retinal hypoxia in long-term diabetic cats. Investigative Ophthalmology & Visual Science. 1998;**39**:1647-1657

[3] Blasiak J, Petrovski G, Vereb Z, Facsko A, Kaarniranta K. Oxidative stress, hypoxia, and autophagy in the neovascular processes of age-related macular degeneration. BioMed Research International. 2014. DOI: 10.1155/2014/768026

[4] Stefánsson E, Geirsdóttir Á, Sigurdsson H. Metabolic physiology in age related macular degeneration. Progress in Retinal and Eye Research. 2011;**30**:72-80. DOI: 10.1016/j.preteyeres.2010.09.003

[5] Arjamaa O, Nikinmaa M, Salminen A, Kaarniranta K. Regulatory role of HIF-1alpha in the pathogenesis of age-related macular degeneration (AMD). Ageing Research Reviews. 2009;**8**:349-358. DOI: 10.1016/j.arr.2009.06.002

[6] Kurihara T, Westenskow PD, Gantner ML, Usui Y, Schultz A, Bravo S, et al. Hypoxia-induced metabolic stress in retinal pigment epithelial cells is sufficient to induce photoreceptor degeneration. eLife. n.d.; **5**. DOI: 10.7554/eLife.14319

[7] Kaur C, Foulds WS, Ling E-A. Hypoxia-ischemia and retinal ganglion cell damage. Clinical Ophthalmology (Auckland, N.Z.). 2008;**2**:879-889

[8] Tezel G, Wax MB. Hypoxia-inducible factor 1alpha in the glaucomatous retina and optic nerve head. Arch Ophthalmol (Chic Ill 1960). 2004;**122**:1348-1356. DOI: 10.1001/archopht.122.9.1348

[9] Hartnett ME, Penn JS. Mechanisms and management of retinopathy of prematurity. The New England Journal of Medicine. 2012;**367**:2515-2526. DOI: 10.1056/NEJMra1208129

[10] Sapieha P, Joyal J-S, Rivera JC, Kermorvant-Duchemin E, Sennlaub F, Hardy P, et al. Retinopathy of prematurity: Understanding ischemic retinal vasculopathies at an extreme of life. The Journal of Clinical Investigation. 2010;**120**:3022-3032. DOI: 10.1172/JCI42142

[11] Di Fiore JM, Kaffashi F, Loparo K, Sattar A, Schluchter M, Foglyano R, et al. The relationship between patterns of intermittent hypoxia and retinopathy of prematurity in preterm infants. Pediatric Research. 2012;**72**:606-612. DOI: 10.1038/pr.2012.132

[12] Holekamp NM, Shui Y-B, Beebe D. Lower intraocular oxygen tension in diabetic patients: Possible contribution to decreased incidence of nuclear sclerotic cataract. American Journal of Ophthalmology. 2006;**141**:1027-1032. DOI: 10.1016/j.ajo.2006.01.016

[13] Arden GB, Sivaprasad S. Hypoxia and oxidative stress in the causation of diabetic retinopathy. Current Diabetes Reviews. 2011;**7**:291-304

[14] Nyengaard JR, Ido Y, Kilo C, Williamson JR. Interactions between hyperglycemia and hypoxia: Implications for diabetic retinopathy. Diabetes. 2004;**53**:2931-2938

[15] Stefánsson E, Machemer R, de Juan E, McCuen BW, Peterson J. Retinal oxygenation and laser treatment in patients with diabetic retinopathy. American Journal of Ophthalmology. 1992;**113**:36-38

[16] Forsythe JA, Jiang BH, Iyer NV, Agani F, Leung SW, Koos RD, et al. Activation of vascular endothelial growth factor gene transcription by hypoxia-inducible factor 1. Molecular and Cellular Biology. 1996;**16**:4604-4613

[17] Wiesener MS, Turley H, Allen WE, Willam C, Eckardt KU, Talks KL, et al. Induction of endothelial PAS domain protein-1 by hypoxia: Characterization and comparison with hypoxia-inducible factor-1alpha. Blood. 1998;**92**:2260-2268

[18] Duan C. Hypoxia-inducible factor 3 biology: Complexities and emerging themes. American Journal of Physiology. Cell Physiology. 2016;**310**:C260-C269. DOI: 10.1152/ajpcell.00315.2015

[19] Zhang P, Yao Q, Lu L, Li Y, Chen P-J, Duan C. Hypoxia-inducible factor 3 is an oxygen-dependent transcription activator and regulates a distinct transcriptional response to hypoxia. Cell Reports. 2014;**6**:1110-1121. DOI: 10.1016/j.celrep.2014.02.011

[20] Appelhoff RJ, Tian Y-M, Raval RR, Turley H, Harris AL, Pugh CW, et al. Differential function of the prolyl hydroxylases PHD1, PHD2, and PHD3 in the regulation of hypoxia-inducible factor. The Journal of Biological Chemistry. 2004;**279**:38458-38465. DOI: 10.1074/jbc.M406026200

[21] Min J-H, Yang H, Ivan M, Gertler F, Kaelin WG, Pavletich NP. Structure of an HIF-1alpha -pVHL complex: Hydroxyproline recognition in signaling. Science. 2002;**296**:1886-1889. DOI: 10.1126/science.1073440

[22] Hon W-C, Wilson MI, Harlos K, Claridge TDW, Schofield CJ, Pugh CW, et al. Structural basis for the recognition of hydroxyproline in HIF-1 alpha by pVHL. Nature. 2002;**417**:975-978. DOI: 10.1038/nature00767

[23] Jaakkola P, Mole DR, Tian YM, Wilson MI, Gielbert J, Gaskell SJ, et al. Targeting of HIF-alpha to the von Hippel-Lindau ubiquitylation complex by O_2-regulated prolyl hydroxylation. Science. 2001;**292**:468-472. DOI: 10.1126/science.1059796

[24] Tanimoto K, Makino Y, Pereira T, Poellinger L. Mechanism of regulation of the hypoxia-inducible factor-1 alpha by the von Hippel-Lindau tumor suppressor protein. The EMBO Journal. 2000;**19**:4298-4309. DOI: 10.1093/emboj/19.16.4298

[25] Lando D, Peet DJ, Whelan DA, Gorman JJ, Whitelaw ML. Asparagine hydroxylation of the HIF transactivation domain a hypoxic switch. Science. 2002;**295**:858-861. DOI: 10.1126/science.1068592

[26] Mowat FM, Luhmann UFO, Smith AJ, Lange C, Duran Y, Harten S, et al. HIF-1alpha and HIF-2alpha are differentially activated in distinct cell populations in retinal ischaemia. PLoS One. 2010;**5**:e11103. DOI: 10.1371/journal.pone.0011103

[27] Ozaki H, Yu AY, Della N, Ozaki K, Luna JD, Yamada H, et al. Hypoxia inducible factor-1alpha is increased in ischemic retina: Temporal and spatial correlation with VEGF expression. Investigative Ophthalmology & Visual Science. 1999;**40**:182-189

[28] Dioum EM, Clarke SL, Ding K, Repa JJ, Garcia JA. HIF-2alpha-haploinsufficient mice have blunted retinal neovascularization due to impaired expression of a proangiogenic gene battery. Investigative Ophthalmology & Visual Science. 2008;**49**:2714-2720. DOI: 10.1167/iovs.07-1469

[29] Koivunen P, Hirsilä M, Remes AM, Hassinen IE, Kivirikko KI, Myllyharju J. Inhibition of hypoxia-inducible factor (HIF) hydroxylases by citric acid cycle intermediates: Possible links between cell metabolism and stabilization of HIF. The Journal of Biological Chemistry. 2007;**282**:4524-4532. DOI: 10.1074/jbc.M610415200

[30] Benzi G, Pastoris O, Dossena M. Relationships between gamma-aminobutyrate and succinate cycles during and after cerebral ischemia. Journal of Neuroscience Research. 1982;**7**:193-201. DOI: 10.1002/jnr.490070210

[31] He W, Miao FJ-P, Lin DC-H, Schwandner RT, Wang Z, Gao J, et al. Citric acid cycle intermediates as ligands for orphan G-protein-coupled receptors. Nature. 2004;**429**:188-193. DOI: 10.1038/nature02488

[32] Li T, Hu J, Du S, Chen Y, Wang S, Wu Q. ERK1/2/COX-2/PGE2 signaling pathway mediates GPR91-dependent VEGF release in streptozotocin-induced diabetes. Molecular Vision. 2014;**20**:1109-1121

[33] Hu J, Li T, Du S, Chen Y, Wang S, Xiong F, et al. The MAPK signaling pathway mediates the GPR91-dependent release of VEGF from RGC-5 cells. International Journal of Molecular Medicine. 2015;**36**:130-138. DOI: 10.3892/ijmm.2015.2195

[34] Sapieha P, Sirinyan M, Hamel D, Zaniolo K, Joyal J-S, Cho J-H, et al. The succinate receptor GPR91 in neurons has a major role in retinal angiogenesis. Nature Medicine. 2008;**14**:1067-1076. DOI: 10.1038/nm.1873

[35] Bek T, Ledet T. Vascular occlusion in diabetic retinopathy. A qualitative and quantitative histopathological study. Acta Ophthalmologica Scandinavica. 1996;**74**:36-40

[36] Schröder S, Palinski W, Schmid-Schönbein GW. Activated monocytes and granulocytes, capillary nonperfusion, and neovascularization in diabetic retinopathy. The American Journal of Pathology. 1991;**139**:81-100

[37] Niki T, Muraoka K, Shimizu K. Distribution of capillary nonperfusion in early-stage diabetic retinopathy. Ophthalmology. 1984;**91**:1431-1439

[38] Hammes H-P, Lin J, Renner O, Shani M, Lundqvist A, Betsholtz C, et al. Pericytes and the pathogenesis of diabetic retinopathy. Diabetes. 2002;**51**:3107-3112

[39] Feit-Leichman RA, Kinouchi R, Takeda M, Fan Z, Mohr S, Kern TS, et al. Vascular damage in a mouse model of diabetic retinopathy: Relation to neuronal and glial changes. Investigative Ophthalmology & Visual Science. 2005;**46**:4281-4287. DOI: 10.1167/iovs.04-1361

[40] Mohr S, Vincent J, Kern T. Minocycline prevents the formation of acellular capillaries in mouse models for diabetic retinopathy. FASEB Journal. 2006;**20**:A1150

[41] Braun RD, Fisher TC, Meiselman HJ, Hatchell DL. Decreased deformability of polymorphonuclear leukocytes in diabetic cats. Microcirculation (New York, N.Y.: 1994). 1996;**3**:271-278

[42] Harris AG, Skalak TC, Hatchell DL. Leukocyte-capillary plugging and network resistance are increased in skeletal muscle of rats with streptozotocin-induced hyperglycemia. International Journal of Microcirculation, Clinical and Experimental. 1994;**14**:159-166

[43] Berkowitz BA, Kowluru RA, Frank RN, Kern TS, Hohman TC, Prakash M. Subnormal retinal oxygenation response precedes diabetic-like retinopathy. Investigative Ophthalmology & Visual Science. 1999;**40**:2100-2105

[44] Behzadian MA, Wang X-L, Shabrawey M, Caldwell RB. Effects of hypoxia on glial cell expression of angiogenesis-regulating factors VEGF and TGF-β. Glia. 1998;**24**:216-225. DOI: 10.1002/(SICI)1098-1136(199810)24:2<216::AID-GLIA6>3.0.CO;2-1

[45] Stone J, Itin A, Alon T, Pe'er J, Gnessin H, Chan-Ling T, et al. Development of retinal vasculature is mediated by hypoxia-induced vascular endothelial growth factor (VEGF) expression by neuroglia. The Journal of Neuroscience. 1995;**15**:4738-4747

[46] Namiki A, Brogi E, Kearney M, Kim EA, Wu T, Couffinhal T, et al. Hypoxia induces vascular endothelial growth factor in cultured human endothelial cells. The Journal of Biological Chemistry. 1995;**270**:31189-31195. DOI: 10.1074/jbc.270.52.31189

[47] Xin X, Rodrigues M, Umapathi M, Kashiwabuchi F, Ma T, Babapoor-Farrokhran S, et al. Hypoxic retinal Muller cells promote vascular permeability by HIF-1-dependent up-regulation of angiopoietin-like 4. Proceedings of the National Academy of Sciences of the United States of America. 2013;**110**:E3425-E3434. DOI: 10.1073/pnas.1217091110

[48] Adamis AP, Miller JW, Bernal MT, D'Amico DJ, Folkman J, Yeo TK, et al. Increased vascular endothelial growth factor levels in the vitreous of eyes with proliferative diabetic retinopathy. American Journal of Ophthalmology. 1994;**118**:445-450

[49] Wang Z, Yadav AS, Leskova W, Harris NR. Attenuation of streptozotocin-induced microvascular changes in the mouse retina with the endothelin receptor A antagonist atrasentan. Experimental Eye Research. 2010;**91**:670-675. DOI: 10.1016/j.exer.2010.08.008

[50] Yadav AS, Harris NR. Effect of tempol on diabetes-induced decreases in retinal blood flow in the mouse. Current Eye Research. 2011;**36**:456-461. DOI: 10.3109/02713683.2011.556300

[51] Lee S, Morgan GA, Harris NR. Ozagrel reverses streptozotocin-induced constriction of arterioles in rat retina. Microvascular Research. 2008;**76**:217-223. DOI: 10.1016/j.mvr.2008.07.005

[52] Wright WS, Harris NR. Ozagrel attenuates early streptozotocin-induced constriction of arterioles in the mouse retina. Experimental Eye Research. 2008;**86**:528-536. DOI: 10.1016/j.exer.2007.12.012

[53] Wright WS, McElhatten RM, Messina JE, Harris NR. Hypoxia and the expression of HIF-1alpha and HIF-2alpha in the retina of streptozotocin-injected mice and rats. Experimental Eye Research. 2010;**90**:405-412. DOI: 10.1016/j.exer.2009.12.002

[54] Wright WS, McElhatten RM, Harris NR. Increase in retinal hypoxia inducible factor-2α, but not hypoxia, early in the progression of diabetes in the rat. Experimental Eye Research. 2011;**93**:437-441. DOI: 10.1016/j.exer.2011.06.003

[55] Wright WS, Singh Yadav A, McElhatten RM, Harris NR. Retinal blood flow abnormalities following six months of hyperglycemia in the Ins2(Akita) mouse. Experimental Eye Research. 2012;**98**:9-15. DOI: 10.1016/j.exer.2012.03.003

[56] Linsenmeier RA. Effects of light and darkness on oxygen distribution and consumption in the cat retina. The Journal of General Physiology. 1986;**88**:521-542

[57] Linsenmeier RA, Braun RD. Oxygen distribution and consumption in the cat retina during normoxia and hypoxemia. The Journal of General Physiology. 1992;**99**:177-197

[58] DY Y, Alder VA, Cringle SJ, EN S, Burns M. Intraretinal oxygen distribution in urethan-induced retinopathy in rats. The American Journal of Physiology. 1998;**274**:H2009-H2017

[59] DY Y, Cringle SJ, Alder V, SEN. Intraretinal oxygen distribution in the rat with graded systemic hyperoxia and hypercapnia. Investigative Ophthalmology & Visual Science. 1999;**40**:2082-2087

[60] D-Y Y, Cringle SJ, E-N S, YPK. Intraretinal oxygen levels before and after photoreceptor loss in the RCS rat. Investigative Ophthalmology & Visual Science. 2000;**41**:3999-4006

[61] Ogawa S, Lee TM, Kay AR, Tank DW. Brain magnetic resonance imaging with contrast dependent on blood oxygenation. Proceedings of the National Academy of Sciences of the United States of America. 1990;**87**:9868-9872

[62] Ogawa S, Lee TM. Magnetic resonance imaging of blood vessels at high fields: In vivo and in vitro measurements and image simulation. Magnetic Resonance in Medicine. 1990;**16**:9-18

[63] Ogawa S, Lee TM, Nayak AS, Glynn P. Oxygenation-sensitive contrast in magnetic resonance image of rodent brain at high magnetic fields. Magnetic Resonance in Medicine. 1990;**14**:68-78

[64] Berkowitz BA, Roberts R, Luan H, Peysakhov J, Mao X, Thomas KA. Dynamic contrast-enhanced mri measurements of passive permeability through blood retinal barrier in diabetic rats. Investigative Ophthalmology & Visual Science. 2004;**45**:2391-2398. DOI: 10.1167/iovs.03-1381

[65] Berkowitz BA, Wilson CA. Quantitative mapping of ocular oxygenation using magnetic resonance imaging. Magnetic Resonance in Medicine. 1995;**33**:579-581. DOI: 10.1002/mrm.1910330419

[66] Duong TQ, Ngan S-C, Ugurbil K, Kim S-G. Functional magnetic resonance imaging of the retina. Investigative Ophthalmology & Visual Science. 2002;**43**:1176-1181

[67] Ito Y, Berkowitz BA. MR studies of retinal oxygenation. Vision Research. 2001;**41**:1307-1311

[68] Falsini B, Riva CE, Logean E. Flicker-evoked changes in human optic nerve blood flow: Relationship with retinal neural activity. Investigative Ophthalmology & Visual Science. 2002;**43**:2309-2316

[69] Petrig BL, Riva CE, Hayreh SS. Laser Doppler flowmetry and optic nerve head blood flow. American Journal of Ophthalmology. 1999;**127**:413-425

[70] Longo A, Geiser M, Riva CE. Subfoveal choroidal blood flow in response to light–dark exposure. Investigative Ophthalmology & Visual Science. 2000;**41**:2678-2683

[71] Hickam JB, Frayser R, Ross JC. A study of retinal venous blood oxygen saturation in human subjects by photographic means. Circulation. 1963;**27**:375-385

[72] Delori FC. Noninvasive technique for oximetry of blood in retinal vessels. Applied Optics. 1988;**27**:1113-1125

[73] Beach JM, Schwenzer KJ, Srinivas S, Kim D, Tiedeman JS. Oximetry of retinal vessels by dual-wavelength imaging: Calibration and influence of pigmentation. Journal of Applied Physiology. 1999;**86**:748-758

[74] Hardarson SH, Harris A, Karlsson RA, Halldorsson GH, Kagemann L, Rechtman E, et al. Automatic retinal Oximetry. Investigative Ophthalmology & Visual Science. 2006;**47**:5011-5016. DOI: 10.1167/iovs.06-0039

[75] Ibrahim MA, Annam RE, Sepah YJ, Luu L, Bittencourt MG, Jang HS, et al. Assessment of oxygen saturation in retinal vessels of normal subjects and diabetic patients with and without retinopathy using flow oximetry system. Quantitative Imaging in Medicine and Surgery. 2015;**5**:86-96. DOI: 10.3978/j.issn.2223-4292.2014.11.26

[76] Lemaillet P, Duncan DD, Lompado A, Ibrahim M, Nguyen QD, Ramella-Roman JC. Retinal spectral imaging and blood flow measurement. Journal of Innovative Optical Health Sciences. 2010;**03**:255-265. DOI: 10.1142/S1793545810001131

[77] Hammer M, Vilser W, Riemer T, Mandecka A, Schweitzer D, Kühn U, et al. Diabetic patients with retinopathy show increased retinal venous oxygen saturation. Graefe's Archive for Clinical and Experimental Ophthalmology. 2009;**247**:1025-1030. DOI: 10.1007/s00417-009-1078-6

[78] Guduru A, Martz TG, Waters A, Kshirsagar AV, Garg S. Oxygen saturation of retinal vessels in all stages of diabetic retinopathy and correlation to ultra-wide field fluorescein angiographyretinal oximetry and IVFA in diabetic retinopathy. Investigative Ophthalmology & Visual Science. 2016;**57**:5278-5284. DOI: 10.1167/iovs.16-20190

[79] Dong Y, Lin L, Yan H, Fu Y, Zong Y, Yuan Y, et al. Shifts in retinal vessel diameter and oxygen saturation in Chinese type 2 diabetes mellitus patients. BMC Ophthalmology. 2016;**16**:43. DOI: 10.1186/s12886-016-0217-1

[80] Jørgensen CM, Hardarson SH, Bek T. The oxygen saturation in retinal vessels from diabetic patients depends on the severity and type of vision-threatening retinopathy. Acta Ophthalmologica. 2014;**92**:34-39. DOI: 10.1111/aos.12283

[81] Jørgensen C, Bek T. Increasing oxygen saturation in larger retinal vessels after photocoagulation for diabetic retinopathy. Investigative Ophthalmology & Visual Science. 2014;**55**:5365-5369. DOI: 10.1167/iovs.14-14811

[82] Khoobehi B, Firn K, Thompson H, Reinoso M, Beach J. Retinal arterial and venous oxygen saturation is altered in diabetic patients. Investigative Ophthalmology & Visual Science. 2013;**54**:7103-7106. DOI: 10.1167/iovs.13-12723

[83] Hardarson SH, Stefánsson E. Retinal oxygen saturation is altered in diabetic retinopathy. The British Journal of Ophthalmology. 2012;**96**:560-563. DOI: 10.1136/bjophthalmol-2011-300640

[84] Jørgensen CM, Bek T. Lack of differences in the regional variation of oxygen saturation in larger retinal vessels in diabetic maculopathy and proliferative diabetic retinopathy.

The British Journal of Ophthalmology. 2017;**101**:752-757. DOI: 10.1136/bjophthalmol-2016-308894

[85] Schweitzer D, Thamm E, Hammer M, Kraft J. A new method for the measurement of oxygen saturation at the human ocular fundus. International Ophthalmology. 2001;**23**:347-353

[86] Schweitzer D, Hammer M, Kraft J, Thamm E, Königsdörffer E, Strobel J. Vivo measurement of the oxygen saturation of retinal vessels in healthy volunteers. IEEE Transactions on Biomedical Engineering. 1999;**46**:1454-1465

[87] Khoobehi B, Beach JM, Kawano H. Hyperspectral imaging for measurement of oxygen saturation in the optic nerve head. Investigative Ophthalmology & Visual Science. 2004;**45**:1464-1472

[88] Yoneya S, Saito T, Nishiyama Y, Deguchi T, Takasu M, Gil T, et al. Retinal oxygen saturation levels in patients with central retinal vein occlusion. Ophthalmology. 2002;**109**:1521-1526

[89] Beach J, Ning J, Khoobehi B. Oxygen saturation in optic nerve head structures by hyperspectral image analysis. Current Eye Research. 2007;**32**:161-170. DOI: 10.1080/02713680601139192

[90] Kashani AH, Kirkman E, Martin G, Humayun MS. Hyperspectral computed tomographic imaging spectroscopy of vascular oxygen gradients in the rabbit retina in vivo. PLoS One. 2011;**6**:e24482. DOI: 10.1371/journal.pone.0024482

[91] Kashani AH, Lopez Jaime GR, Saati S, Martin G, Varma R, Humayun MS. Noninvasive assessment of retinal vascular oxygen content among normal and diabetic human subjects: A study using hyperspectral computed tomographic imaging spectroscopy. Retina (Philadelphia, Pa.). 2014;**34**:1854-1860. DOI: 10.1097/IAE.0000000000000146

[92] Vanderkooi JM, Maniara G, Green TJ, Wilson DF. An optical method for measurement of dioxygen concentration based upon quenching of phosphorescence. The Journal of Biological Chemistry. 1987;**262**:5476-5482

[93] Wilson DF, Rumsey WL, Green TJ, Vanderkooi JM. The oxygen dependence of mitochondrial oxidative phosphorylation measured by a new optical method for measuring oxygen concentration. The Journal of Biological Chemistry. 1988;**263**:2712-2718

[94] Knopp JA, Longmuir IS. Intracellular measurement of oxygen by quenching of fluorescence of pyrenebutyric acid. Biochimica et Biophysica Acta (BBA) - General Subjects. 1972;**279**:393-397. DOI: 10.1016/0304-4165(72)90158-4

[95] Shonat RD, Wilson DF, Riva CE, Pawlowski M. Oxygen distribution in the retinal and choroidal vessels of the cat as measured by a new phosphorescence imaging method. Applied Optics. 1992;**31**:3711-3718. DOI: 10.1364/AO.31.003711

[96] Shonat RD, Wilson DF, Riva CE, Cranstoun SD. Effect of acute increases in intraocular pressure on intravascular optic nerve head oxygen tension in cats. Investigative Ophthalmology & Visual Science. 1992;**33**:3174-3180

[97] Blumenröder S, Augustin AJ, Koch FH. The influence of intraocular pressure and systemic oxygen tension on the intravascular pO2 of the pig retina as measured with phosphorescence imaging. Survey of Ophthalmology. 1997;**42**(Suppl 1):S118-S126

[98] Shonat RD, Kight AC. Frequency Domain Imaging of Oxygen Tension in the Mouse Retina. Oxyg. Transp. Boston, MA: Tissue XXIII. Springer; 2003. pp. 243-247. DOI: 10.1007/978-1-4615-0205-0_40

[99] Shonat RD, Kight AC. Oxygen tension imaging in the mouse retina. Annals of Biomedical Engineering. 2003;**31**:1084-1096

[100] Wilson DF, Vinogradov SA, Grosul P, Vaccarezza MN, Kuroki A, Bennett J. Oxygen distribution and vascular injury in the mouse eye measured by phosphorescence-lifetime imaging. Applied Optics. 2005;**44**:5239-5248

[101] Wilson DF, Vinogradov SA, Grosul P, Kuroki A, Bennett J. Imaging Oxygen Pressure in the Retina of the Mouse Eye. Oxyg. Transp. Boston, MA: Tissue XXVI, Springer; 2005. pp. 159-165. DOI: 10.1007/0-387-26206-7_22

[102] Shahidi M, Shakoor A, Blair NP, Mori M, Shonat RD. A method for chorioretinal oxygen tension measurement. Current Eye Research. 2006;**31**:357-366. DOI: 10.1080/02713680600599446

[103] Shakoor A, Gupta M, Blair NP, Shahidi M. Chorioretinal vascular oxygen tension in spontaneously breathing anesthetized rats. Ophthalmic Research. 2007;**39**:103-107. DOI: 10.1159/000099246

[104] Shakoor A, Blair NP, Mori M, Shahidi M. Chorioretinal vascular oxygen tension changes in response to light flicker. Investigative Ophthalmology & Visual Science. 2006;**47**:4962-4965. DOI: 10.1167/iovs.06-0291

[105] Shahidi M, Wanek J, Blair NP, Little DM, Wu T. Retinal tissue oxygen tension imaging in the rat. Investigative Ophthalmology & Visual Science. 2010;**51**:4766-4770. DOI: 10.1167/iovs.09-4710

[106] Felder AE, Wanek J, Tan MR, Blair NP, Shahidi M. A method for combined retinal vascular and tissue oxygen tension imaging. Scientific Reports. 2017;**7**:10622. DOI: 10.1038/s41598-017-10955-1

[107] Mezu-Ndubuisi OJ, Teng P, Wanek J, Blair NP, Chau FY, Reddy NM, et al. In vivo retinal vascular oxygen tension imaging and fluorescein angiography in the mouse model of oxygen-induced retinopathy. Investigative Ophthalmology & Visual Science. 2013;**54**:6968-6972. DOI: 10.1167/iovs.13-12126

[108] Buerk DG, Tsai AG, Intaglietta M, Johnson PC. Comparing Tissue PO2 Measurements by Recessed Microelectrode and Phosphorescence Quenching. Oxyg. Transp. Boston, MA: Tissue XX, Springer; 1998. pp. 367-374. DOI: 10.1007/978-1-4615-4863-8_44

[109] Gross MW, Karbach U, Groebe K, Franko AJ, Mueller-Klieser W. Calibration of misonidazole labeling by simultaneous measurement of oxygen tension and labeling density in multicellular spheroids. International Journal of Cancer. 1995;**61**:567-573

[110] Raleigh JA, Miller GG, Franko AJ, Koch CJ, Fuciarelli AF, Kelly DA. Fluorescence immunohistochemical detection of hypoxic cells in spheroids and tumours. British Journal of Cancer. 1987;**56**:395-400

[111] Miller GG, Best MW, Franko AJ, Koch CJ, Raleigh JA. Quantitation of hypoxia in multicellular spheroids by video image analysis. International Journal of Radiation Oncology. 1989;**16**:949-952. DOI: 10.1016/0360-3016(89)90893-6

[112] Chapman JD, Franko AJ, Sharplin J. A marker for hypoxic cells in tumours with potential clinical applicability. British Journal of Cancer. 1981;**43**:546-550

[113] Varia MA, Calkins-Adams DP, Rinker LH, Kennedy AS, Novotny DB, Fowler WC, et al. Pimonidazole: A novel hypoxia marker for complementary study of tumor hypoxia and cell proliferation in cervical carcinoma. Gynecologic Oncology. 1998;**71**:270-277. DOI: 10.1006/gyno.1998.5163

[114] Franko AJ, Chapman JD. Binding of 14C-misonidazole to hypoxic cells in V79 spheroids. British Journal of Cancer. 1982;**45**:694-699

[115] Aguilera KY, Brekken RA. Hypoxia studies with pimonidazole in vivo. Bio-Protocol. 2014;**4**

[116] Ly A, Yee P, Vessey KA, Phipps JA, Jobling AI, Fletcher EL. Early inner retinal astrocyte dysfunction during diabetes and development of hypoxia, retinal stress, and neuronal functional loss. Investigative Ophthalmology & Visual Science. 2011;**52**:9316-9326. DOI: 10.1167/iovs.11-7879

[117] Rothschild P-R, Salah S, Berdugo M, Gélizé E, Delaunay K, Naud M-C, et al. ROCK-1 mediates diabetes-induced retinal pigment epithelial and endothelial cell blebbing: Contribution to diabetic retinopathy. Scientific Reports. 2017;**7**:8834. DOI: 10.1038/s41598-017-07329-y

[118] Curtis TM, Gardiner TA, Stitt AW. Microvascular lesions of diabetic retinopathy: Clues towards understanding pathogenesis? Eye (London, England). 2009;**23**:1496-1508. DOI: 10.1038/eye.2009.108

[119] Gooyer de TE, Stevenson KA, Humphries P, Simpson DAC, Gardiner TA, Stitt AW. Retinopathy is reduced during experimental diabetes in a mouse model of outer retinal degeneration. Investigative Ophthalmology & Visual Science. 2006;**47**:5561-5568. DOI: 10.1167/iovs.06-0647

[120] Evans SM, Kim K, Moore CE, Uddin MI, Capozzi ME, Craft JR, et al. Molecular probes for imaging of hypoxia in the retina. Bioconjugate Chemistry. 2014;**25**:2030-2037. DOI: 10.1021/bc500400z

[121] Uddin MI, Evans SM, Craft JR, Marnett LJ, Uddin MJ, Jayagopal A. Applications of azo-based probes for imaging retinal hypoxia. ACS Medicinal Chemistry Letters. 2015;**6**:445-449. DOI: 10.1021/ml5005206

[122] Myochin T, Hanaoka K, Komatsu T, Terai T, Nagano T. Design strategy for a near-infrared fluorescence probe for matrix metalloproteinase utilizing highly cell permeable

boron dipyrromethene. Journal of the American Chemical Society. 2012;**134**:13730-13737. DOI: 10.1021/ja303931b

[123] Kiyose K, Hanaoka K, Oushiki D, Nakamura T, Kajimura M, Suematsu M, et al. Hypoxia-sensitive fluorescent probes for in vivo real-time fluorescence imaging of acute ischemia. Journal of the American Chemical Society. 2010;**132**:15846-15848. DOI: 10.1021/ja105937q

[124] Uddin MI, Evans SM, Craft JR, Capozzi ME, McCollum GW, Yang R, et al. *In Vivo* imaging jof retinal hypoxia in a model of oxygen-induced retinopathy. Scientific Reports. 2016;**6**:srep31011. DOI: 10.1038/srep31011

[125] Uddin MI, Jayagopal A, McCollum GW, Yang R, Penn JS. In vivo imaging of retinal hypoxia using HYPOX-4-dependent fluorescence in a mouse model of laser-induced retinal vein occlusion (RVO). Investigative Ophthalmology & Visual Science. 2017;**58**:3818-3824. DOI: 10.1167/iovs.16-21187

[126] Joussen AM, Poulaki V, Le ML, Koizumi K, Esser C, Janicki H, et al. A central role for inflammation in the pathogenesis of diabetic retinopathy. FASEB journal : official publication of the Federation of American Societies for Experimental Biology. 2004;**18**:1450-1452. DOI: 10.1096/fj.03-1476fje

[127] Zheng L, Gong B, Hatala DA, Kern TS. Retinal ischemia and reperfusion causes capillary degeneration: Similarities to diabetes. Investigative Ophthalmology & Visual Science. 2007;**48**:361-367. DOI: 10.1167/iovs.06-0510

[128] Simpson DA, Murphy GM, Bhaduri T, Gardiner TA, Archer DB, Stitt AW. Expression of the VEGF gene family during retinal vaso-obliteration and hypoxia. Biochemical and Biophysical Research Communications. 1999;**262**:333-340. DOI: 10.1006/bbrc.1999.1201

[129] Kernt M, Thiele S, Liegl RG, Kernt B, Eibl K, Haritoglou C, et al. Axitinib modulates hypoxia-induced blood-retina barrier permeability and expression of growth factors. Growth factors (Chur, Switzerland). 2012;**30**:49-61. DOI: 10.3109/08977194.2011.639300

[130] Tiedeman JS, Kirk SE, Srinivas S, Beach JM. Retinal oxygen consumption during hyperglycemia in patients with diabetes without retinopathy. Ophthalmology. 1998;**105**:31-36

Section 3

Proliferative Diabetic Retinopathy

Proliferative Diabetic Retinopathy: An Overview of Vitreous Immune and Biomarkers

Andi Arus Victor and Ratna Sitompul

Additional information is available at the end of the chapter

http://dx.doi.org/10.5772/intechopen.74366

Abstract

This chapter discusses about the effect of vitreous immune system and biomarkers on the progression of proliferative diabetic retinopathy. Immune system and biomarkers have been believed to have an important role in the progression of diabetic retinopathy (DR) severity. Hyperglycemic will influence immune cells resulting in chronic inflammation on the retina. This condition progressively disrupts the blood-retinal barrier in retina causing those inflammatory molecules and immune cells to transfer from circulation. The transfer of these molecules plays an important part in the progression of proliferative diabetic retinopathy. In addition, biomarkers are indicators for some complex processes happened in our body, and are measured to determine diagnosis and prognosis of some treatment. There are several biomarkers that have been identified in DR patients including biomarkers of oxidative stress, hypoxia-inducible factors, angiogenic factors, pro-inflammatory cytokines, chemokines, cell adhesion molecules, and soluble CD200. The value of these biomarkers will tell us their possible role in the progression of DR. By improving the knowledge of molecular pathway in DR pathophysiology, the advancement of selective therapy approaches could be discovered and the management of DR could be more efficient.

Keywords: biomarker, diabetic retinopathy, hyperglycemia, immune system, inflammation

1. Introduction

Diabetic retinopathy (DR) is the most common chronic microvascular complication of uncontrolled diabetes mellitus leading to preventable blindness. Diabetic retinopathy is often classified based on its severity into mild non-proliferative diabetic retinopathy (NPDR), moderate

NPDR, severe NPDR, and proliferative diabetic retinopathy (PDR) [1–3]. The major risk factors for developing DR are the duration of diabetes, hyperglycemia, hypertension, and dyslipidemia [4]. Glucose concentration increases in retinal cells leading to saccular capillary microaneurysms, pericyte deficient capillaries, and degenerate capillaries that decrease the retinal perfusion and contribute to the progression of DR [4]. Several types of evidence prove the benefits of tight glycemic and blood pressure control in decelerating the progression of DR. Nevertheless, the numbers of DR patients and the development of DR complications are still increasing, while therapeutic approaches are limited [1, 2].

For the last several decades, many studies have been performed in order to better understand DR progression from a molecular viewpoint. The biochemical mechanisms implicated in DR progression have been shown in various animal models and patients with diabetes [1]. It is believed that the involvement of hyperglycemia and hormonal factors in diabetic patients could disturb hemostasis in the retina and change the balance of some mediators including growth factors, cytokines, inflammatory, and adhesion molecules [5]. These changes result in altered capillary permeability, apoptosis of capillary cells, and angiogenesis, leading to DR complications [3]. With improved clarity of molecular pathways in DR pathophysiology, the advancement of selective therapeutic approaches could be discovered and the management of DR could be more effective [1, 5]. This chapter focuses on the inflammatory molecules and biomarkers involved in the pathophysiology of DR.

2. The immune system in proliferative diabetic retinopathy

The immune system protects the body from both exogenous pathogens called pathogen-associated molecular patterns (PAMPs) and endogenous harmful molecules known as damage-associated molecular patterns (DAMPs). DAMPs include oxidized or glycated proteins, mislocated proteins/antigens, and intracellular contents released by necrotic cells. In normal conditions, the immune system regulates the inflammatory process and prevents uncontrolled inflammation that damages cells. In hyperglycemic conditions, the accumulation of DAMPs induces chronic inflammation in various tissues, which in turn manifests into the various complications of diabetes, including diabetic retinopathy [6].

The retina is one of few tissues in the human body that has immune privilege. It is protected from the attack of the systemic immune system by a series of complex defense mechanisms. This protection is afforded by a physical barrier formed between endothelial cells of retinal vasculature as the inner blood-retinal barrier (BRB) and retinal pigmented epithelial cells as the outer BRB. This barrier limits the movement of cells and molecules from the systemic circulation into the retinal parenchyma. The BRB also separates retinal antigens within the intraocular compartment, avoiding activation of T cells. This phenomenon is known as immunological ignorance. In addition, there is no lymphatic system in the retina. This inhibits systemic immune cells from detecting damage-associated molecular patterns in the retina thus preventing an overt systemic inflammatory response. Retinal cells (retinal neurons and RPE cells) express immune modulators that can suppress immune cells and complement system activation. The retina is protected by the local innate immune system (microglia, perivascular macrophages, and the complement system) whose activation is tightly controlled [6].

The immune system plays an important role in the progression of DR. Under hyperglycemic conditions, over activation of the innate immune system takes place, resulting in chronic inflammation of the retina. A study by Urbančič et al. showed the presence of T lymphocytes in the vitreous of patients with PDR. They found that the CD4/CD8 lymphocyte ratio in vitreous is higher compared to the blood ratio in these PDR patients, demonstrating the presence of a local inflammatory process [7]. Prolonged local inflammation in hyperglycemic conditions in the retina may develop into a chronic inflammatory response that is detrimental to the integrity of BRB [6, 8–10]. The destruction of the barrier shifts the retina from its "privileged state" when the BRB functions normally to "compromised state" when the BRB has broken down. Complement system activation also increases in diabetic conditions and this dysregulated activation is known to be involved in the degeneration of retinal vessels. Dysfunctional barriers permit inflammatory molecules and immune cells from systemic circulation to enter the retina and cause further deterioration of the tissue [6, 11]. Cytological examination of the vitreous samples from PDR patients were found to contain significant amounts of macrophages suggesting the infiltration of systemic immune cells into the retina [12, 13]. In addition, there was an increase in adhesion molecule expression and pro-inflammatory cytokine production, suggesting the role of defective neutrophil activity in the development of chronic inflammation in diabetic retinopathy [14, 15] (**Figure 1**).

3. Vitreous biomarkers in proliferative diabetic retinopathy

A biomarker is an objective measurement that is evaluated as an indicator for some complex processes happening in our body [16]. Biomarkers are usually measured to determine the diagnosis and prognosis of some treatments [17]. There are several biomarkers that can be found in diabetic retinopathy patients including biomarkers of oxidative stress, hypoxia-inducible factors, angiogenic factors, pro-inflammatory cytokines, chemokines, cell adhesion molecules, and CD200. The value of these biomarkers tells us their possible role in the progression of diabetic retinopathy [5, 6, 18–21] (**Figure 2**).

3.1. Biomarkers of oxidative stress

The presence of oxidative stress biomarkers indicate an imbalance of reactive oxygen species (ROS) and the functional capabilities of cellular antioxidants [18, 22]. This imbalance can cause

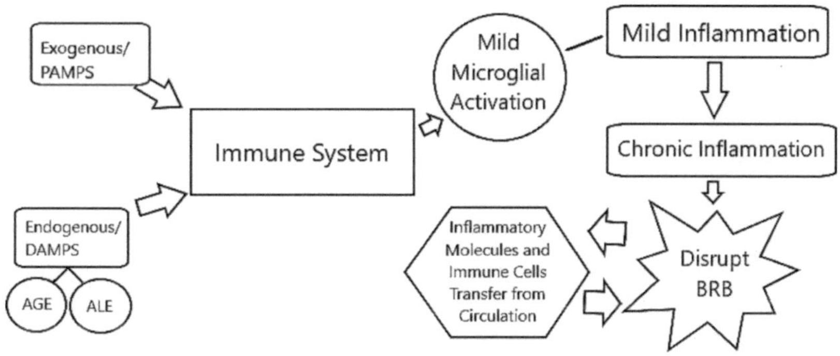

Figure 1. Immune system role in progression of diabetic retinopathy.

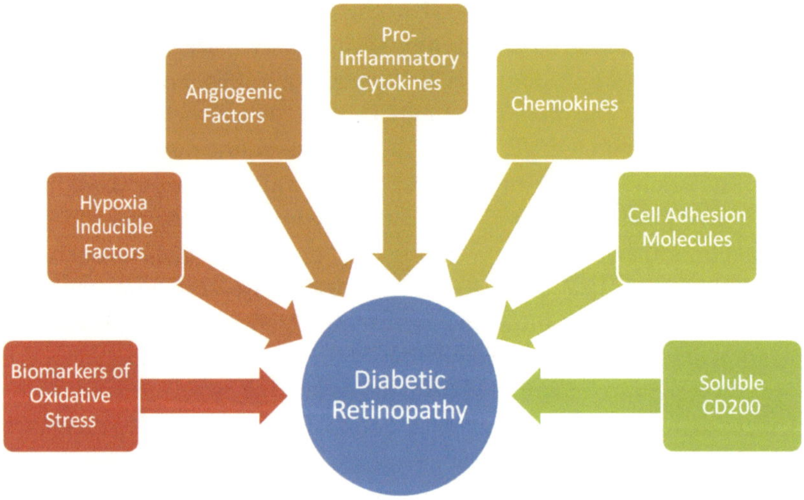

Figure 2. Vitreous biomarkers involved in proliferative diabetic retinopathy.

cell instability and contribute to the development of many diseases, including diabetic retinopathy [18, 23]. Oxidative stress will remain high even after the patient reaches a normoglycemic state. This phenomenon is called "metabolic memory" and can lead to the accumulation of ROS in diabetic patients [24]. The biological markers of oxidative stress can include changes in molecules of the antioxidant system and molecules modified by ROS. Antioxidant enzymes like the superoxide dismutases are an example of changes in molecules of the antioxidant system, and malondialdehyde is the best known oxidative stress marker [18].

3.1.1. Superoxide dismutases

Superoxide dismutases (SODs) are a group of enzymes found in our cells, which function as major antioxidant defense systems against ROS in the body. SODs consist of three isoforms: the cytoplasmic Cu/ZnSOD (SOD1), the mitochondrial MnSOD (SOD2), and the extracellular Cu/ZnSOD (SOD3), all of which require catalytic metal (Cu or Mn) to activate. SOD activities will increase due to the presence of oxidative stress in the body. Vitreous SOD activity can also be used to measure oxidative stress levels inside the eye, allowing it to be a viable biomarker of oxidative stress in patients with PDR. Brzović-Šarić et al. state that PDR patients serum oxidative stress markers were higher than non-diabetic patients with an eye disorders (NDED) serum. Brzović-Šarić et al. found a mean activity level of SODs in the vitreous of male diabetic patients at 30.5 ± 2.5 U/mL, and 28.5 ± 3.8 U/mL in vitreous of female patients with diabetes [25]. Our previous study found a mean activity level of SODs in vitreous of patients with PDR at 0.403 + 0.50 U/mL [26].

3.1.2. Malondialdehyde

Malondialdehyde (MDA) is a highly reactive compound produced by lipid peroxidation of polyunsaturated lipid found in cell membranes. MDA exerts its oxidative stress effect inside cells and forms molecules called advanced lipoxidation end-products (ALE). MDA levels in specific tissues can be measured to represent oxidative damage induced by physical or chemical oxidative stress in the corresponding tissues [24, 25, 27]. Brzović-Šarić et al. found a significant difference between vitreous MDA values in non-diabetic patients with an eye disorder and PDR patients [25]. On the other hand, several studies found an increase in MDA serum of diabetic patients compared to control patients, but there was no significant difference in MDA serum level between non-proliferative DR and proliferative DR patients [24, 27]. Our study found a mean activity level of MDA in the vitreous of patients with PDR at 1.661 ± 1.21 nmol/mL [26]. Another study about oxidative stress levels with PDR by Mancino et al. found a mean activity level of MDA in vitreous of patients with PDR at 520 ± 210 nmol/mL [24]. What causes these differences in vitreous MDA levels still needs to be explored.

3.2. Hypoxia-inducible factors

HIF-1α is a DNA-binding protein complex that is continuously expressed and degraded by cells in the body. Under hypoxic conditions, the HIF-1α degradation rate decreases, causing increased concentration of HIF-1α which then translocates into the nucleus and dimerizes with HIF-1β. The HIF-1 complex then regulates the expression of genes responsible for the hypoxic response of the cell by binding into the hypoxia response element (HRE) [28]. The HIF-1 complex is known to cause angiogenic effects on these hypoxic tissues [29]. Previous studies by Arden et al. on patients with diabetic retinopathy shows that hypoxia is present in retinal tissues suffering from oxidative damage [30]. Accordingly, Wang and co-workers found increased levels of HIF-1α protein in vitreous samples of PDR patients compared to levels in non-diabetic subjects [28]. Furthermore, the vitreous levels of vascular endothelial growth factor (VEGF) and HIF-1α were highly correlated in PDR patients. Several studies demonstrated positive immunohistochemical staining for HIF-1α and VEGF proteins in epiretinal neurovascular membranes. This evidence shows that HIF might play an important role in regulating the neovascularization of retina in PDR [31, 32].

3.3. Angiogenic factors

Angiogenesis is a complex multistep process that involves angiogenic factors and is induced by various cytokines and growth factors [33]. These factors have been suggested to be correlated with the development of diabetic retinopathy [5, 33–35]. These are also known to be hypoxia-responsive factors [5, 35]. Pro-angiogenic factors, like VEGF, angiopoientin, and erythropoietin are well-known factors contributing to neovascularization and whose levels increase in diabetic retinopathy patients [3, 5, 33–35]. Several therapies designed to target these factors have been proven effective in decreasing the progression of the disease [5].

3.3.1. Vascular endothelial growth factor

Vascular endothelial growth factor (VEGF) is a signaling molecule that promotes development of new blood vessels. It is released by cells in response to hypoxic conditions. Abcouwer stated that VEGF increases vascular permeability by promoting the disassembly of junctions between endothelial cells. This leakage can cause diabetic macular edema

(DME) [5]. Several studies have shown marked increases of VEGF in vitreous and vitreous compared to plasma concentration in DME and PDR patients [19, 36–46]. Treatments that target VEGF have been proven highly effective in treating DR. VEGF antibodies, which were originally used for cancer treatments, such as bevacizumab and its correlate ranibizumab have been used effectively. These have also been tested in several small trials which showed improved vision in DR patients, demonstrating the involvement of VEGF in the pathophysiology of PDR [5, 36].

Brzović-Šarić also demonstrated a significant difference between vitreous VEGF values in non-diabetic patients with eye disorders and PDR patients [25]. Loukovaara et al. state that VEGF is a major factor in PDR development and found significant increases of VEGF levels in the vitreous of DR patients (465.1 ± 1470.2 pg/mL) compared to control patients (40.3 ± 165.8 pg/mL) [37]. Our study found a mean level of VEGF in vitreous of patients with PDR of 0.356 + 0.60 pg/mL [26]. Yoshimura et al. found that there was significantly elevated VEGF in PDR patients, but not in DME patients [47]. The increased levels of VEGF expression in patients with diabetic retinopathy was mainly produced by Muller glial cells. Experiments in diabetic mice, demonstrated that conditional knockout of VEGF in Muller cells effectively blocked the increase in retinal VEGF expression [48]. Lange and co-workers suggest that oxygen tension levels were positively correlated with vitreous VEGF levels, and oxygen tension levels at the posterior pole were increased in PDR patients [49]. The vitreous levels of VEGF will decrease in the most severe stage of PDR, when there is a transition from angiogenesis to fibrosis [50].

3.3.2. Angiopoietin

Angiopoietins are a group of proteins with the role of regulating vascular development and angiogenesis. Two types of angiopoietins, angiopoietin-1 and angiopoietin-2, contribute to the maintenance of retinal vasculature. The former exerts a stabilizing effect on vessels, organizing and limiting the angiogenesis response, while the latter exhibits angiogenic activity if VEGF is present, but promotes endothelial cell death and vascular regression in the absence of VEGF. The ratio between these two angiopoietins represents the inflammatory process in the cell. Fiedler et al. state that hypoxia/ischemia activates endothelial cells upregulating angiopoientin-2 thus lowering the angiopoientin-1/angiopoientin-2 ratio [37, 51]. A recent publication by Loukovaara et al. demonstrates significant correlation between intravitreal concentrations of Ang-2 with MMP-9, VEGF, EPO and TGFb1 levels in diabetic eyes undergoing vitrectomy, indicating its role in retinal tissue neovascularization in PDR patients. The study shows a slight increase in angiopoietin-1 from the control group (19.1 ± 25.4 pg/mL) to the study group (25.6 ± 27.1 pg/mL), and a great increase in angiopoietin-2 from the control group (43.0 ± 60.9 pg/mL) to the study group (317.1 ± 419.1 pg/mL), thus lowering the angiopoietin-1/angiopoietin-2 ratio in study group. The plasma value of angiopoietin-1 is similar in both groups, but the plasma value of angiopoietin-2 is increased from the control group (2623.4 ± 2142.0 pg/mL) compared to the study group (5690.4 ± 8064.7 pg/mL) [36, 37, 52]. Several studies state that angiopoietin-1 can be used for the prevention and treatment of diabetic retinopathy by its ability to suppress VEGF expression in diabetic retina [53].

http://dx.doi.org/10.5772/intechopen.74366

3.3.3. Erythropoietin

Erythropoietin (EPO) is a glycoprotein cytokine that acts as a major regulator of erythropoiesis. Besides erythropoiesis, several studies state that erythropoietin has a neuroprotective and angiogenic effect in brain and retina. Production of EPO in serum and vitreous is mainly caused by hypoxia [54–57]. EPO is found in many organs, including kidney, liver, brain, and retina [55]. The angiogenic effect of EPO is a potential equivalent to VEGF, and has been suspected as an important factor in the angiogenesis of PDR [56]. Watanabe et al. showed that vitreous EPO levels of PDR patients are significantly higher (464.0 mlU/mL) compared to non-diabetic patients (36.5 mlU/mL). They also found that EPO levels are higher with active as compared to quiescent PDR [54]. These are consistent with Katsura et al., who also reported increases of vitreous EPO levels in PDR patients compared to controls [55]. Cristina et al. found that EPO levels in vitreous fluid are significantly higher (326 mU/mL) compared to serum EPO (11.2 mU/mL) in PDR patients [56]. This shows that intraocular production is responsible for the high concentration of erythropoietin found in the vitreous fluid of retinal degeneration patients [54, 56, 57]. Garci et al. found increased vitreous EPO concentrations in DME patients (430 mU/mL) compared to control patients (25 mU/mL) [57]. Treatment involving the erythropoietin blockade is likely to be beneficial, but may worsen the disease due to the decrease of its neuroprotective function [54].

3.3.4. Matrix metalloproteinases 9

Matrix metalloproteinases (MMPs) are a family of zinc ion-binding endopeptidases that degrade most of the extracellular matrix (ECM). MMPs regulate many cellular functions including apoptosis, wound healing, and angiogenesis. In angiogenesis, MMPs increase VEGF production and remove physical barriers to new vessel growth [58, 59]. MMPs are produced as a response to increased oxidative stress. Diabetic patients often have increased MMP, mainly MMP-9 and MMP-2 in the retina and vitreous. These are controlled by endogenous tissue inhibitors of metalloproteinases (TIMPs). TIMP-1 regulates MMP-9 and TIMP-2 regulates MMP-2 [59]. Several studies suggest that MMPs are responsible for many diabetic complications, including cardiomyopathy, nephropathy, and retinopathy. MMPs are suspected to facilitate apoptosis of retinal capillary cells during early stages leading to disruption of blood-retinal barrier integrity [58–60]. Kowluru et al. found an increase in MMP-9 and a decrease in TIMP-1 in the retina of DR patients [58]. Abu et al. found significant increases in vitreous zymography levels of MMP-9 in PDR patients (392.3 ± 253.6 scanning units) compared to non-diabetic control patients (168.2 ± 65.0 scanning units). However, the levels of vitreous MMP-2 in PDR patients (540.9 ± 185.6 scanning units) did not differ significantly from non-diabetic control patients (505.4 ± 216.1 scanning units) [60]. Inhibitors of MMPs have been used to treat several diseases, however, there have been no studies using these inhibitors to treat DR patients [59].

3.3.5. Transforming growth factor β

Transforming growth factor β (TGF-β) is a polypeptide responsible for controlling cell proliferation and differentiation. It is usually secreted in a latent phase and must be transformed to become a mature active form. In the human eye, there are three known TGF-β isoforms (TGF-β_1, TGF-β_2, and TGF-β_3), where the posterior segment of the eye mainly contains TGF-β_2 as the dominant form [61–63]. Hirase et al. found an increase in total vitreous TGF-β_2 levels in PDR patients (2634 ± 1652 pg/mL) compared to control patients (1305 ± 972 pg/mL) [61]. This result is also consistent with a McAuley et al. study about vitreous biomarkers in diabetic retinopathy [62]. The mature active form of TGF-β_2 levels are also increased in PDR patients. This increase correlates with the disease severity, suggesting that TGF-β_2 angiogenesis properties play a role in the progression of PDR [61].

3.4. Pro-inflammatory cytokines

Pro-inflammatory cytokines are usually secreted by inflammatory cells in response to hypoxia or hyperglycemia [64]. Well-known pro-inflammatory cytokines, such as tumor necrosis factor, interleukin, interferon, and receptor tyrosine kinase are found to be elevated in the vitreous of diabetic retinopathy patients, suggesting their important role in the pathogenesis of this disease [5, 64, 65]. Cytokines can induce the progression of diabetic retinopathy directly and indirectly. Direct mechanisms include the direct engagement with target cells to induce neovascularization [64]. While indirect mechanisms induce leukocytes and endothelial cells to produce pro-angiogenic mediators, which in turn induce neovascularization [64, 65]. Therapy targeting these cytokines may be beneficial, but we need better understanding about the cytokine roles to do so [5].

3.4.1. Tumor necrosis factor-α

Tumor necrosis factors-α (TNF-α), a pro-inflammatory cytokine, is primarily synthesized by macrophages and T cells. Its expression is regulated by NF-κβ and it has been associated with the pathogenesis of several chronic inflammatory diseases including type 2 diabetes. Its function is primarily as an immune-modulator and it also plays a role in neovascularization and fibroplasia [3]. Costagliola et al. suggest that TNF-α is a potent mediator of leukostasis and contributes to blood-retinal barrier breakdown [3, 66]. TNF-α concentration is found elevated in the vitreous of PDR patients and the vitreous/serum ratio of TNF-α is also found higher compared to non-diabetic patients. Costagliola et al. found that TNF-α levels were lower in controls (1.9 pg/mL) than the PDR group (13.5 pg/mL) and increased with the severity of the disease [3, 66]. TNF-α has a short half-life (~4 min), making its analyzation prone to producing false negative results. Soluble TNF-α receptors (sTNF-α-Rs) have a longer half-life, making it a more reliable marker of the activation of TNF-α system [29, 31, 67–71].

3.4.2. Interleukin

Several studies have shown that there is involvement of interleukins in the development of PDR. The most common interleukins found in DR patients are IL-6 and IL-8, where their concentrations were found increased in the vitreous of patients with PDR and prolonged hyperglycemia [3, 42, 47, 72–82]. Their role in the pathogenesis of PDR is still under investigation but evidence suggests the possibility of a rather direct contribution. IL-6 controls immune cells responses by shifting T-helper cell populations, inhibiting the production of Th1 cells, promoting the differentiation of Th2 and Th17 cells, and infiltration of monocytes and T cells [9, 10, 83].

In vitro study of IL-6 reports its ability to increase endothelial cell and vascular cell permeability by rearranging actin filaments and by changing the shape of endothelial cells [3, 65]. Several studies state that IL-6 also plays an important role in angiogenesis by activating VEGF, and regulating expression of metalloproteinases [3, 64]. IL-8 is known to be a potent angiogenic factor and also a potent chemoattractant and activator of neutrophils and T lymphocytes [64, 84, 85]. Increase of IL-8 concentrations in PDR patients, suggest that they are upregulated in response to oxygen stress and contribute to triggering inflammatory reactions. Study by Takahashi et al. shows that there is a significant increase in IL-6 and IL-8 values in PDR patients (918.0 and 2168.0 ng/mL) compared to control patient (517.0 and 343.0 ng/mL) [85]. Elner et al. also found increased levels of IL-8 in active PDR patients (24.7 ± 4.5 ng/mL) compared to control patients (7.5 ± 2.3 ng/mL), however inactive PDR patients (11.6 ± 5.2 ng/mL) did not differ significantly from controls [79]. It is most likely that VEGF expression causes an increase of IL-8 [86]. On the other hand, IL-10 concentration is not increased in the vitreous of patients with PDR. IL-10 is another important immunoregulatory cytokine that is induced by cell hypoxia. IL-10 activates nitric oxide and increases vascular permeability during the development of PDR [3, 65, 84, 85].

3.4.3. Monokine induced by interferon-γ

Monokine induced by interferon-γ (Mig) attracts activated T cells and has potent angiostatic activity. Several studies suggest that Mig correlates with VEGF and contributes to the progression of neovascularization in DR patients. The main function of Mig in the progression of DR might be related to its leukostasis function [88, 89]. Wakabayashi et al. found significant increases in vitreous concentration of Mig in active (148 pg/mL) and inactive (82.3 pg/mL) DR patients compared with non-diabetic patients who had macular disease (21 pg/mL). However, there was no significant difference in serum Mig concentration between DR patients (85.9 pg/mL) and control subjects (70.4 pg/mL) [87]. Takeuchi et al. also found an increase in Mig vitreous concentration in PDR patients compared to epiretinal membrane patients, idiopathic macular hole patients, and uveitis patients [88].

3.4.4. Receptor tyrosine kinase

Receptor tyrosine kinase (c-kit) is expressed by bone marrow and involved in intracellular signaling. It plays an important role in cell proliferation, cell adhesion, cell survival, and neovascularization [89]. Several studies have shown that C-kit plays an important role in the angiogenic process of PDR. C-kit has a soluble form called s-kit that can be generated by proteolytic cleavage [90]. Abu et al. found an increase of c-kit expression in membranes from patients with active neovascularization (697.4 ± 1528.1 pg/mL) compared to patients with inactive PDR (205.3 ± 106.4 pg/mL) and control patients (87.5 ± 91.5 pg/mL). This demonstrates that an increase of c-kit expression is correlated to the progression of PDR [90]. However, Lee et al. found a slight decrease of c-kit values in the PDR group compared to NPDR group [91].

3.5. Chemokine

Chemokines are low molecular weight proteins that have many functions, including enhanced immune responses, regulation of homeostasis, and controlling angiogenesis [20, 92, 93].

Chemokines are often referred to as secondary pro-inflammatory mediators, whose activation is induced by pro-inflammatory cytokines or primary pro-inflammatory mediators. Chemokines induce a specific leukocyte type and can bind to chemokine-receptors on target cells [20, 92]. Chemokines are usually categorized into two groups, the CXC group is chemotactic for neutrophils and the CC group is chemotactic for monocytes and lymphocytes [20, 92]. Several studies show an increase of chemokines in vitreous of PDR patients, suggesting that they have roles in mediating angiogenesis and fibrosis in PDR patients [20, 93, 94]. Struyf et al. stated that chemokines have different roles based on disease progression. In the early phase, chemokines can induce leukocyte attraction and in late phase, they can induce neovascularization [93]. Das et al. introduced a new therapy targeting chemokines in patients with DME [94].

3.5.1. Monocyte chemotactic protein-1

Monocyte chemotactic protein-1 (MCP-1) is a member of the chemokine group which is responsible for regulating migration and infiltration of monocyte/macrophages to the site of inflammation, making MCP-1 a pro-inflammatory cytokine that plays a central role in CNS inflammation [2]. Hyun et al. stated that MCP-1 is a major cause of vascular complications in diabetes [95]. It is also a potent inducer of angiogenesis and fibrosis. MCP-1 levels were found elevated in the vitreous of diabetic patients and their levels are higher than serum [2, 97]. Ning et al. stated that advanced glycation end product (AGE) stimulation activates retinal neurons to release MCP-1 activating retinal microglial cells. Their study also shows a progressive increase of MCP-1 along with the progression of disease, indicating it may be an important link in diabetic retinopathy pathogenesis [2, 96]. Hyperglycemia also has been shown to increase MCP-1 expression from retinal vascular endothelial cells, RPE cells, and Muller glial cells [2, 97]. Reddy et al. demonstrated significantly higher levels of MCP-1 in PDR patients compared to normal glucose tolerance (NGT) patients. MCP-1 is also steadily increased along with the progression of PDR [97].

3.5.2. Interferon gamma-induced protein-10

Interferon gamma-induced protein-10 (IP-10), also known as CXCL10, is one of the CXC chemokine members. CXC chemokine has unique properties in which it can act as either an angiogenic or angiostatic factor, depending on the protein configuration of the molecule. IP-10 is inducible directly or through activation of IFN-γ, TNF-α, NFkB, viruses, or microbial products. Boulday et al. reported that VEGF induced the expression of IP-10 [1]. IP-10 binds CXCR3 receptors inducing apoptosis, angiostasis, and chemotaxis. It has been suggested that IP-10 is associated with inflammatory diseases including immune dysfunction and infectious disease. This protein has also been proposed to be involved in the pathophysiology of diabetic retinopathy, especially in the development of neovascularization. Elner et al. found a significant increase in the level of IP-10 in patients with PDR compared to the patients with non-diabetic eye diseases (NDED; 11.7 ± 1.1 ng/mL and 4.6 ± 0.9 ng/mL; $p < 0.001$, CI 95%). They also assumed that pan-retinal laser photocoagulation (PRP) might influence elevated IP-10 levels. The exact mechanism of the PRP-induced IP-10 involution of PDR remains to be elucidated [79].

3.5.3. Stromal cell-derived factor-1

Stromal cell-derived factor-1 (SDF-1) is a chemokine with a major role in the ischemic damage repair process. It recruits endothelial progenitor cells (EPCs) from the bone marrow to the site of repair and upregulates expression of VEGF, increasing the angiogenic process. This pro-angiogenic factor is categorized as being hypoxia-responsive and is found to be upregulated in PDR [98–100]. Chen et al. found that vitreous concentrations of SDF-1 and VEGF are correlated in eyes with PDR. They also found that vitreous levels of SDF-1 are significantly higher in PDR patients (306.37 ± 134.25 pg/mL) than in patients with idiopathic macular hole (86.91 ± 55.05 pg/mL) [101]. Butler et al. demonstrate an increase of SDF-1 concentration in the vitreous of patients with PDR and this increase correlates directly with disease severity. They also demonstrated that intravitreal injection of triamcinolone dramatically decreased the concentration of vitreal VEGF and SDF-1, suggesting it as another possible treatment for PDR [98].

3.5.4. High-mobility group box-1

High-mobility group box-1 (HMGB1) is a nonhistone DNA-binding protein that facilitates transcription. HMGB1 can be released into the extracellular space by active secretion from certain cells such as activated monocytes and macrophages, mature dendritic cells, natural killer cells, and endothelial cells. Necrotic cell death can also cause passive leakage of HMGB1 from the nucleus as the protein is no longer bound to DNA. HMGB1 can bind to the receptor for advanced glycation end products (RAGE) and toll-like receptor 2 (TLR-2), where it acts as a pro-inflammatory cytokine, activating NF-κβ resulting in the overexpression of other pro-inflammatory molecules such as TNF-α, MCP-1, and ICAM-1 [41, 102, 103]. El-Asrar et al. demonstrated a significant correlation between neovascularization levels in epiretinal membranes of patients with PDR and the expression of HMGB1 and RAGE [41]. Yao Yu et al. also found an increase of HMGB1 concentration in the vitreous of PDR patients. This increase in vitreous happens in the later phases of DR, and differs from other inflammatory cytokines. They also found increases of RAGE protein and decreases of TLR-2 protein in DR rats, suggesting that the involvement of HMGB-1 is mainly through its binding with RAGE [102].

3.6. Cell adhesion molecules

Adhesion molecules have many roles in our body, including embryology, immunology, and malignancy [21]. Several studies show increases of these molecules in PDR patients, suggesting that cell to cell interaction plays a major role in the development of PDR [79, 104–106]. These molecules regulate lymphocyte recruitment to vascular endothelium. Well-known adhesion molecules found in PDR patients are intercellular adhesion molecule-1 (ICAM-1) and vascular cell adhesion molecules-1 (VCAM-1), which are required for initiation of adhesion-dependent immune response [21, 106].

3.6.1. Intercellular adhesion molecule-1

Intercellular adhesion molecule-1 (ICAM-1), also known as CD54, is a cell surface glycoprotein encoded by the ICAM1 gene. ICAM-1 is usually expressed on the surface of endothelial cells and cells of the immune system. It works as a cell adhesion molecule that recruits nearby circulating leukocytes to the inflamed location. In PDR patients, ICAM-1 is suspected as one of the deteriorating factors, promoting leukostasis and inflammation on nearby retinal tissue. Several experiments show leukostasis as a possible mechanism in diabetic retinal vasculature injury. Cells which are attached, mainly granulocytes and monocytes cause microvascular occlusion and capillary injury [106]. Leukostasis in DR is mainly caused by endothelial activation and increased surface expression of intercellular adhesion molecules (ICAM-1) [107]. Hillier et al. stated that increases in ICAM-1 correlate with the severity of DR in patients [108]. Our study on ICAM-1 showed an increase of ICAM-1 expression in PDR patients with more than 10 years of diabetes history [103]. Yan et al. in their study about the effects of intravitreal ranibizumab injection on ICAM-1 levels in PDR patients, demonstrated a decrease of ICAM-1 levels a week after intravitreal injection [109].

3.6.2. Vascular cell adhesion molecule-1

Vascular cell adhesion molecule-1 (VCAM-1) is an immunoglobulin supergene family of cellular adhesion molecules that are involved in the transmigration of monocytes, eosinophils, and lymphocytes [105, 110–112]. Oxidative stress, VEGF, and hypercholesterolemia increase the expression of VCAM-1 in the brain and retina [111, 113, 114]. It is released by endothelial cells and is present as an early feature of inflammatory disease [111, 113]. Several studies state that VCAM-1 promotes angiogenesis in PDR patients [105, 112–114]. Burgos et al. demonstrated increases in vitreous concentration of VCAM-1 in PDR patients (26 ng/mL) compared to non-diabetic patients in whom a vitrectomy was performed (22 ng/mL) [104]. These results are also consistent with Mroczek et al. in their study about the influence of glucose control on the activation of the intraocular molecular system [114]. There are also reports of increase VCAM-1 concentration in the retinal vessels and serum of PDR patients [111, 112].

3.7. Soluble CD200

CD200 is a novel immunosuppressive molecule found in neuronal cells. CD200 exists in a cell membrane-bound form and a soluble form. It exerts inhibitory effects on microglia/macrophages via interaction with the CD200 receptor (CD200R) [115]. DR-related neuronal degeneration also reduces CD200 concentration and further induces microglial activation [6]. Recent study on CD200 revealed that levels of sCD200 in vitreous of patients with PDR are significantly higher compared to that in the vitreous of patients without PDR. Xu et al. showed increases in mean sCD200 levels in the PDR group (182 ± 17.63 pg/mL) compared to non-diabetic patients with other conditions who requires pars plana vitrectomy (56.86 ± 6.573 pg/mL). This study also showed that vitreous levels of sCD200 are higher in PDR patients with DME (266.9 ± 28.82 pg/mL) or traction retinal detachment (TRD) (256.9 ± 34.50 pg/mL) compared to PDR patients without DME (136.9 ± 15.13 pg/mL) or TRD (146.9 ± 15.97 pg/mL). sCD200 level increases also have significant statistical correlations with the increase of several angiogenic and inflammatory molecules such as VEGF, IL-6, IL-8 and IL-10 [115].

Acknowledgements

This article's publication is partially supported by the United States Agency for International Development (USAID) through the Sustainable Higher Education Research Alliance (SHERA) Program for Universitas Indonesia's Scientific Modeling, Application, Research and Training for City-centered Innovation and Technology (SMART CITY) Project, Grant #AID-497-A-1600004, Sub Grant #IIE-00000078-UI-1.

Conflict of interest

There are no conflicts of interest in this chapter.

Author details

Andi Arus Victor* and Ratna Sitompul

*Address all correspondence to: arvimadao@yahoo.com

Department of Ophthalmology, Faculty of Medicine, Universitas Indonesia, Cipto Mangunkusumo National General Hospital, Jakarta, Indonesia

References

[1] Simó-Servat O, Hernández C, Simó R. Usefulness of the vitreous fluid analysis in the translational research of diabetic retinopathy. Mediators of Inflammation. 2012;**2012**:872978. DOI: 10.1155/2012/872978

[2] Dong N et al. Upregulation of retinal neuronal MCP-1 in the rodent model of diabetic retinopathy and its function in vitro. Investigative Ophthalmology & Visual Science. 2012; **53**:7567. DOI: 10.1167/iovs.12-9446

[3] Paine SK et al. Association of tumor necrosis factor α, interleukin 6, and interleukin 10 promoter polymorphism with proliferative diabetic retinopathy in type 2 diabetic subjects. Retina. 2012;**32**:1197-1203. DOI: 10.1097/IAE.0b013e31822f55f3

[4] Lü H. Inflammation and diabetic retinopathy. Diabetic Retinopathy. 2012;**1**:125-136. DOI: 10.5772/28635

[5] Abcouwer SF. Angiogenic factors and cytokines in diabetic retinopathy. Journal of Clinical & Cellular Immunology. 2013;**11**:1. DOI: 10.4172/2155-9899

[6] Xu H, Chen M. Diabetic retinopathy and dysregulated innate immunity. Vision Research. 2017;**139**:39-46. DOI: 10.1016/j.visres.2017.04.013

[7] Urbančič M, Kloboves Prevodnik V, Petrovič D, Globočnik Petrovič M. A flow cytometric analysis of vitreous inflammatory cells in patients with proliferative diabetic retinopathy. BioMed Research International. 2013;**2013**:1-7. DOI: 10.1155/2013/251528

[8] Khandelwal PJ, Herman AM, Moussa CEH. Inflammation in the early stages of neurodegenerative pathology. Journal of Neuroimmunology. 2011;**238**:1-11. DOI: 10.1016/j.jneuroim.2011.07.002

[9] Holm TH, Draeby D, Owens T. Microglia are required for astroglial toll-like receptor 4 response and for optimal TLR2 and TLR3 response. Glia. 2012;**60**:630-638. DOI: 10.1002/glia.22296

[10] Graeber MB, Li W, Rodriguez ML. Role of microglia in CNS inflammation. FEBS Letters. 2011;**585**:3798-3805. DOI: 10.1016/j.febslet.2011.08.033

[11] Bresgen M, Baum U, Esser P, Wiedemann P, Heimann K. Protein composition of the vitreous body in proliferative diabetic retinopathy. An analysis with 2-D-electrophoresis. Der Ophthalmologe. 1994;**91**:758-762. PMID: 7849428

[12] Canataroglu H et al. Interleukin (IL)-6, interleukin (IL)-8 levels and cellular composition of the vitreous humor in proliferative diabetic retinopathy, proliferative vitreoretinopathy, and traumatic proliferative vitreoretinopathy. Ocular Immunology and Inflammation. 2005;**13**:375-381. DOI: 10.1080/09273940490518900

[13] Cutler CW, Eke P, Arnold RR, Van Dyke TE. Defective neutrophil function in an insulin-dependent diabetes mellitus patient. A case report. Journal of Periodontology. 1991;**62**:394-401. DOI: 10.1902/jop.1991.62.6.394

[14] Bouma G, Lam-Tse WK, Wierenga-Wolf AF, Drexhage HA, Versnel MA. Increased serum levels of MRP-8/14 in type 1 diabetes induce an increased expression of CD11b and an enhanced adhesion of circulating monocytes to fibronectin. Diabetes. 2004;**53**:1979-1986. DOI: 10.2337/diabetes.53.8.1979

[15] Hatanaka E, Monteagudo PT, Marrocos MSM, Campa A. Neutrophils and monocytes as potentially important sources of proinflammatory cytokines in diabetes. Clinical and Experimental Immunology. 2006;**146**:443-447. DOI: 10.1111/j.1365-2249.2006.03229.x

[16] Zhang R et al. Association between myeloperoxidase levels and risk of coronary artery disease. JAMA: The Journal of the American Medical Association. 2001;**286**:2136-2142. DOI: 10.1001/jama.286.17.2136

[17] Ho E, Karimi Galougahi K, Liu C-C, Bhindi R, Figtree GA. Biological markers of oxidative stress: Applications to cardiovascular research and practice. Redox Biology. 2013; **1**:483-491. DOI: 10.1016/j.redox.2013.07.006

[18] Zelen I et al. Antioxidant enzymes activities and plasma levels of oxidative stress markers in B-chronic lymphocytic leukemia patients. Journal of BUON. 2010;**15**:330-336. PMID: 20658731

[19] Nawaz MI et al. Autocrine CCL2, CXCL4, CXCL9 and CXCL10 signal in retinal endothelial cells and are enhanced in diabetic retinopathy. Experimental Eye Research. 2013;**109**:67-76. DOI: 10.1016/j.exer.2013.01.008

[20] Abu El-Asrar AM, Struyf S, Kangave D, Geboes K, Van Damme J. Chemokines in proliferative diabetic retinopathy and proliferative vitreoretinopathy. European Cytokine Network. 2006;**17**:155-165. PMID: 17194635

[21] Etzioni A. Adhesion molecules-their role in health and disease. Pediatric Research. 1996; **39**:191-198. DOI: 10.1203/00006450-199602000-00001

[22] Pandey KB, Rizvi SI. Markers of oxidative stress in erythrocytes and plasma during aging in humans. Oxidative Medicine and Cellular Longevity. 2010;**3**:2-12. DOI: 10.4161/oxim.3.1.10476

[23] Kowluru RA, Chan PS. Oxidative stress and diabetic retinopathy. Experimental Diabetes Research. 2007;**43603**:1-12. DOI: 10.1155/2007/43603

[24] Mancino R et al. Lipid peroxidation and total antioxidant capacity in vitreous, aqueous humor, and blood samples from patients with diabetic retinopathy. Molecular Vision. 2011;**17**:1298-1304. PMID: 21633716

[25] Brzović-Šarić V et al. Levels of selected oxidative stress markers in the vitreous and serum of diabetic retinopathy patients. Molecular Vision. 2015;**21**:649-664. PMID: 26120270

[26] Victor AA et al. Effect of laser photocoagulation and bevacizumab intravitreal in proliferative diabetic retinopathy: Review on biomarkers of oxidative stress. Medical Journal of Indonesia. 2014;**23**:79-86. DOI: http://dx.doi.org/10.13181/mji.v23i2.756

[27] Dave A, Kalra P, Gowda BHR, Krishnaswamy M. Association of bilirubin and malondialdehyde levels with retinopathy in type 2 diabetes mellitus. Indian Journal of Endocrinology and Metabolism. 2015;**19**:373-377. DOI: 10.4103/2230-8210.152777

[28] Greer SN, Metcalf JL, Wang Y, Ohh M. The updated biology of hypoxia-inducible factor. EMBO Journal. 2012;**31**:2448-2460. DOI: 10.1038/emboj.2012.125

[29] Weidemann A, Johnson RS. Biology of HIF-1α. Cell Death and Differentiation. 2008; **15**:621-627. DOI: 10.1038/cdd.2008.12

[30] Arden GB, Sivaprasad S. Hypoxia and oxidative stress in the causation of diabetic retinopathy. Current Diabetes Reviews. 2011;**7**:291-304. PMID: 21916837

[31] Han XX, Guo CM, Li Y, Hui YN. Effects of bevacizumab on the neovascular membrane of proliferative diabetic retinopathy: Reduction of endothelial cells and expressions of VEGF and HIF-1α. Molecular Vision. 2012;**18**:1-9. PMID: 22232563

[32] Abu El-Asrar AM, Missotten L, Geboes K. Expression of hypoxia-inducible factor-1alpha and the protein products of its target genes in diabetic fibrovascular epiretinal membranes. The British Journal of Ophthalmology. 2007;**91**:822-826. DOI: 10.1136/bjo.2006.109876

[33] Noma H et al. Regulation of angiogenesis in diabetic retinopathy: Possible balance between vascular endothelial growth factor and endostatin. Archives of Ophthalmology (Chicago, Ill. 1960). 2002;**120**:1075-1080. PMID: 12149062

[34] Praidou A et al. Angiogenic growth factors and their inhibitors in diabetic retinopathy. Current Diabetes Reviews. 2010;**6**:304-312. DOI: BSP/CDR/E-Pub/00029

[35] Crawford TN, Alfaro DV, Kerrison JB, Jablon EP. Diabetic retinopathy and angiogenesis. Current Diabetes Reviews. 2009;**5**:8-13. DOI: 10.2174/157339909787314149

[36] Watanabe D et al. Vitreous levels of angiopoietin 2 and vascular endothelial growth factor in patients with proliferative diabetic retinopathy. American Journal of Ophthalmology. 2005;**139**:476-481. DOI: 10.1016/j.ajo.2004.10.004

[37] Loukovaara S et al. Ang-2 upregulation correlates with increased levels of MMP-9, VEGF, EPO and TGFβ1 in diabetic eyes undergoing vitrectomy. Acta Ophthalmologica. 2013;**91**:531-539. DOI: 10.1111/j.1755-3768.2012.02473.x

[38] Aiello LP et al. Vascular endothelial growth factor in ocular fluid of patients with diabetic retinopathy and other retinal disorders. New England Journal of Medicine. 1994;**331**:1480-1487. DOI: 10.1056/NEJM199412013312203

[39] Abu El-Asrar AM et al. Angiogenesis regulatory factors in the vitreous from patients with proliferative diabetic retinopathy. Acta Diabetologica. 2013;**50**:545-551. DOI: 10.1007/s00592-011-0330-9

[40] Zhou J, Wang S, Xia X. Role of intravitreal inflammatory cytokines and angiogenic factors in proliferative diabetic retinopathy. Current Eye Research. 2012;**37**:416-420. DOI: 10.3109/02713683.2012.661114

[41] El-Asrar AMA et al. High-mobility group box-1 and biomarkers of inflammation in the vitreous from patients with proliferative diabetic retinopathy. Molecular Vision. 2011; **17**:1829-1838. PMID: 21850157

[42] Funatsu H et al. Vitreous levels of interleukin-6 and vascular endothelial growth factor are related to diabetic macular edema. Ophthalmology. 2003;**110**:1690-1696. DOI: 10.1016/S0161-6420(03)00568-2

[43] Wakabayashi Y et al. Correlation of vascular endothelial growth factor with chemokines in the vitreous in diabetic retinopathy. Retina. 2010;**30**:339-344. DOI: 10.1097/IAE.0b013e3181bd2f44

[44] Mohan N, Monickaraj F, Balasubramanyam M, Rema M, Mohan V. Imbalanced levels of angiogenic and angiostatic factors in vitreous, plasma and postmortem retinal tissue of patients with proliferative diabetic retinopathy. Journal of Diabetes and its Complications. 2012;**26**:435-441. DOI: 10.1016/j.jdiacomp.2012.05.005

[45] Wang X, Wang G, Wang Y. Intravitreous vascular endothelial growth factor and hypoxia-inducible factor 1a in patients with proliferative diabetic retinopathy. American Journal of Ophthalmology. 2009;**148**:883-889. DOI: 10.1016/j.ajo.2009.07.007

[46] Wakabayashi Y et al. Persistent overproduction of intraocular vascular endothelial growth factor as a cause of late vitreous hemorrhage after vitrectomy for proliferative diabetic retinopathy. Retina. 2017;**1**:2317-2325. DOI: 10.1097/IAE.0000000000001490

[47] Yoshimura T et al. Comprehensive analysis of inflammatory immune mediators in vitreoretinal diseases. PLoS One. 2009;**4**:8158. DOI: 10.1371/journal.pone.0008158

[48] Wang J, Xu X, Elliott MH, Zhu M, Le YZ. Müller cell-derived VEGF is essential for diabetes-induced retinal inflammation and vascular leakage. Diabetes. 2010;**59**:2297-2305. DOI: 10.2337/db09-1420

[49] Lange CAK et al. Intraocular oxygen distribution in advanced proliferative diabetic retinopathy. American Journal of Ophthalmology. 2011;**152**:406-412. DOI: 10.1016/j.ajo.2011.02.014

[50] Kuiper EJ et al. The angio-fibrotic switch of VEGF and CTGF in proliferative diabetic retinopathy. PLoS One. 2008;**3**:2675. DOI: 10.1371/journal.pone.0002675

[51] Fiedler U, Augustin HG. Angiopoietins: A link between angiogenesis and inflammation. Trends in Immunology. 2006;**27**:552-558. DOI: 10.1016/j.it.2006.10.004

[52] Huber M, Wachtlin J. Vitreous levels of proteins implicated in angiogenesis are modulated in patients with retinal or choroidal neovascularization. Ophthalmologica. 2012;**228**:188-193. DOI: 10.1159/000339952

[53] Joussen AM et al. Suppression of diabetic retinopathy with angiopoietin-1. The American Journal of Pathology. 2002;**160**:1683-1693. DOI: 10.1016/S0002-9440(10)61115-7

[54] Watanabe D et al. Erythropoietin as a retinal angiogenic factor in proliferative diabetic retinopathy. New England Journal of Medicine. 2005;**353**:782-792. DOI: 10.1056/NEJMoa041773

[55] Katsura Y et al. Erythropoietin is highly elevated in vitreous fluid of patients with proliferative diabetic retinopathy. Diabetes Care. 2005;**28**:2252-2254. DOI: 10.2337/DIACARE.28.9.2252

[56] Hernández C et al. Erythropoietin is expressed in the human retina and it is highly elevated in the vitreous fluid of patients with diabetic macular edema. Diabetes Care. 2006;**29**:2028-2033. DOI: 10.2337/dc06-0556

[57] Garcí-Arumí J et al. Vitreous levels of erythropoietin in patients with macular oedema secondary to retinal vein occlusions: A comparative study with diabetic macular oedema. Eye. 2009;**23**:1066-1071. DOI: 10.1038/eye.2008.230

[58] Kowluru RA. Role of matrix metalloproteinase-9 in the development of diabetic retinopathy and its regulation by H-Ras. Investigative Ophthalmology & Visual Science. 2010;**51**:4320-4326. DOI: 10.1167/iovs.09-4851

[59] Kowluru RA, Zhong Q, Santos JM. Matrix metalloproteinases in diabetic retinopathy: Potential role of MMP-9. Expert Opinion on Investigational Drugs. 2012;**21**:797-805. DOI: 10.1517/13543784.2012.681043

[60] Abu El-Asrar AM et al. Relationship between vitreous levels of matrix metalloproteinases and vascular endothelial growth factor in proliferative diabetic retinopathy. PLoS One. 2012;**8**:85857. DOI: 10.1371/journal.pone.0085857

[61] Hirase K et al. Transforming growth factor β2 in the vitreous in proliferative diabetic retinopathy. Archives of Ophthalmology. 1998;**116**:738. DOI: 10.1001/archopht.116.6.738

[62] McAuley AK et al. Vitreous biomarkers in diabetic retinopathy: A systematic review and meta-analysis. Journal of Diabetes and its Complications. 2014;**28**:419-425. DOI: 10.1016/j.jdiacomp.2013.09.010

[63] Gacka M, Adamiec J. The role of transforming growth factor-beta in the pathogenesis of diabetic retinopathy. Przegląd Lekarski. 2006;**63**:296-298. PMID: 17036509

[64] Semeraro F et al. Diabetic retinopathy: Vascular and inflammatory disease. Journal of Diabetes Research. 2015;**2015**:582060. DOI: 10.1155/2015/582060

[65] Murugeswari P, Al E. Proinflammatory cytokines and angiogenic and anti-angiogenic factors in vitreous of patients with proliferative diabetic retinopathy and eales' disease. Retina. 2008;**28**:817-824. DOI: 10.1097/IAE.0b013e31816576d5

[66] Costagliola C et al. TNF-alpha levels in tears: A novel biomarker to assess the degree of diabetic retinopathy. Mediators of Inflammation. 2013;**2013**:629529. DOI: 10.1155/2013/629529

[67] Koleva-Georgieva DN, Sivkova NP, Terzieva D. Serum inflammatory cytokines IL-1beta, IL-6, TNF-alpha and VEGF have influence on the development of diabetic retinopathy. Folia Medica (Plovdiv). 2011;**53**:44-50. PMID: 21797106

[68] Myśliwiec M et al. The role of vascular endothelial growth factor, tumor necrosis factor alpha and interleukin-6 in pathogenesis of diabetic retinopathy. Diabetes Research and Clinical Practice. 2008;**79**:141-146. DOI: 10.1016/j.diabres.2007.07.011

[69] Doganay S et al. Comparison of serum NO, TNF-alpha, IL-1beta, sIL-2R, IL-6 and IL-8 levels with grades of retinopathy in patients with diabetes mellitus. Eye (London, England). 2002;**16**:163-170. DOI: 10.1038/sj/EYE/6700095

[70] Gustavsson C, Agardh E, Bengtsson B, Agardh C D. TNF-α is an independent serum marker for proliferative retinopathy in type 1 diabetic patients. Journal of Diabetes and its Complications. 2008;**22**(5):22309-22316. DOI: 10.1016/j.jdiacomp.2007.03.001

[71] Ben-Mahmud BM et al. Clinical validation of a link between TNF-α and the glycosylation enzyme core 2 GlcNAc-T and the relationship of this link to diabetic retinopathy. Diabetologia. 2006;**49**:2185-2191. DOI: 10.1007/s00125-006-0332-2

[72] Funatsu H et al. Aqueous humor levels of cytokines are related to vitreous levels and progression of diabetic retinopathy in diabetic patients. Graefe's Archive for Clinical and Experimental Ophthalmology. 2005;**243**:3-8. DOI: 10.1007/s00417-004-0950-7

[73] Gustavsson C, Agardh CD, Agardh E. Profile of intraocular tumour necrosis factor-α and interleukin-6 in diabetic subjects with different degrees of diabetic retinopathy. Acta Ophthalmologica. 2013;**91**:445-452. DOI: 10.1111/j.1755-3768.2012.02430.x

[74] Lee WJ, Kang MH, Seong M, Cho HY. Comparison of aqueous concentrations of angiogenic and inflammatory cytokines in diabetic macular oedema and macular oedema due to branch retinal vein occlusion. British Journal of Ophthalmology. 2012;**96**:1426-1430. DOI: 10.1136/bjophthalmol-2012-301913

[75] Schoenberger SD et al. Increased prostaglandin E2 (PGE_2) levels in proliferative diabetic retinopathy, and correlation with VEGF and inflammatory cytokines. Investigative Ophthalmology and Visual Science. 2012;**53**:5906. DOI: 10.1167/iovs.12-10410

[76] Kauffmann DJ et al. Cytokines in vitreous humor: Interleukin-6 is elevated in proliferative vitreoretinopathy. Investigative Ophthalmology and Visual Science. 1994;**35**:900-906. DOI: 10.1167/iovs.12-10410

[77] Yuuki T et al. Inflammatory cytokines in vitreous fluid and serum of patients with diabetic vitreoretinopathy. Journal of Diabetes and its Complications. 2001;**15**:257-259. DOI: 10.1016/S1056-8727(01)00155-6

[78] Adamiec-Mroczek J, Oficjalska-Młyńczak J. Assessment of selected adhesion molecule and proinflammatory cytokine levels in the vitreous body of patients with type 2 diabetes — Role of the inflammatory–immune process in the pathogenesis of proliferative diabetic retinopathy. Graefe's Archive for Clinical and Experimental Ophthalmology. 2008;**246**:1665-1670. DOI: 10.1007/s00417-008-0868-6

[79] Elner SG et al. Cytokines in proliferative diabetic retinopathy and proliferative vitreoretinopathy. Current Eye Research. 1995;**14**:1045-1053. PMID: 8585935

[80] Fonollosa A et al. Vitreous levels of interleukine-8 and monocyte chemoattractant protein-1 in macular oedema with branch retinal vein occlusion. Eye. 2010;**24**:1284-1290. DOI: 10.1038/eye.2009.340

[81] Umazume K et al. Effects of soluble CD14 and cytokine levels on diabetic macular edema and visual acuity. Retina. 2013;**33**:1020-1025. DOI: 10.1097/IAE.0b013e31826f0688

[82] Rincon M. Interleukin-6: From an inflammatory marker to a target for inflammatory diseases. Trends in Immunology. 2012;**33**:571-577. DOI: 10.1016/j.it.2012.07.003

[83] Ghasemi H, Ghazanfari T, Yaraee R, Faghihzadeh S, Hassan ZM. Roles of IL-8 in ocular inflammations: A review. Ocular Immunology and Inflammation. 2011;**19**:401-412. DOI: 10.3109/09273948.2011.618902

[84] Taub DD, Anver M, Oppenheim JJ, Longo DL, Murphy WJ. T lymphocyte recruitment by interleukin-8 (IL-8). IL-8-induced degranulation of neutrophils releases potent chemoattractants for human T lymphocytes both in vitro and in vivo. Journal of Clinical Investigation. 1996;**97**:1931-1941. DOI: 10.1172/JCI118625

[85] Takahashi S, Adachi K, Suzuki Y, Maeno A, Nakazawa M. Profiles of inflammatory cytokines in the vitreous fluid from patients with rhegmatogenous retinal detachment and their correlations with clinical features. BioMed Research International. 2016;**2016**:1-9. DOI: 10.1155/2016/4256183

[86] Lee TH, Avraham H, Lee SH, Avraham S. Vascular endothelial growth factor modulates neutrophil transendothelial migration via up-regulation of interleukin-8 in human brain microvascular endothelial cells. Journal of Biological Chemistry. 2002;**277**:10445-10451. DOI: 10.1074/jbc.M107348200

[87] Wakabayashi Y et al. Increased levels of monokine induced by interferon-γ (Mig) in the vitreous of patients with diabetic retinopathy. Diabetic Medicine. 2008;**25**:875-877. DOI: 10.1111/j.1464-5491.2008.02466.x

[88] Takeuchi M et al. Elevated levels of cytokines associated with th2 and th17 cells in vitreous fluid of proliferative diabetic retinopathy patients. PLoS One. 2015;**10**:e0137358. DOI: 10.1371/journal.pone.0137358

[89] Ray P, Krishnamoorthy N, Ray A. Emerging functions of c-kit and its ligand stem cell factor in dendritic cells. Cell Cycle. 2008;**7**:2826-2832. DOI: 10.4161/cc.7.18.6752

[90] Abu El-Asrar AM, Nawaz MI, Kangave D, Mairaj Siddiquei M, Geboes K. Angiogenic and vasculogenic factors in the vitreous from patients with proliferative diabetic retinopathy. Journal of Diabetes Research. 2013;**2013**:539658. DOI: 10.1155/2013/539658

[91] Lee IG, Chae SL, Kim JC. Involvement of circulating endothelial progenitor cells and vasculogenic factors in the pathogenesis of diabetic retinopathy. Eye. 2006;**20**:546-552. DOI: 10.1038/sj.eye.6701920

[92] Dai Y, Wu Z, Wang F, Zhang Z, Yu M. Identification of chemokines and growth factors in proliferative diabetic retinopathy vitreous. BioMed Research International. 2014;**2014**: 1-9. DOI: 10.1155/2014/486386

[93] Struyf S et al. Role of chemokines in diabetic retinopathy. Acta Ophthalmologica. 2015;**93**:1-8. DOI: 10.1111/j.1755-3768.2015.0221

[94] Das A. Inflammatory chemokines: A novel target in early diabetic retinopathy. National Institute of Health. 2015;**1**:1-10

[95] Jeon HJ, Choi HJ, Park BH, Lee YH, Oh T. Association of monocyte chemoattractant protein-1 (MCP-1) 2518A/G polymorphism with proliferative diabetic retinopathy in korean type 2 diabetes. Yonsei Medical Journal. 2013;**54**:621. DOI: 10.3349/ymj.2013.54.3.621

[96] Abu el-Asrar AM et al. Monocyte chemotactic protein-1 in proliferative vitreoretinal disorders. American Journal of Ophthalmology. 1997;**123**:599-606. PMID: 9152065

[97] Reddy S et al. Association of increased levels of MCP-1 and cathepsin-D in young onset type 2 diabetes patients (T2DM-Y) with severity of diabetic retinopathy. Journal of Diabetes and its Complications. 2017;**31**:804-809. DOI: 10.1016/j.jdiacomp.2017.02.017

[98] Butler JM et al. SDF-1 is both necessary and sufficient to promote proliferative retinopathy. Journal of Clinical Investigation. 2005;**115**:86-93. DOI: 10.1172/JCI22869

[99] Brooks HL et al. Vitreous levels of vascular endothelial growth factor and stromal-derivedfactor 1 in patients with diabetic retinopathy and cystoid macular edema beforeand after intraocular injection of triamcinolone. Journal of Clinical Investigation. 2004;**122**:1801. DOI: 10.1172/JCI22869

[100] Campochiaro PA. Ocular neovascularization. Angiogenesis: An Integrative Approach from Science to Medicine. 2013;**91**:311-321. DOI: 10.1007/978-0-387-71518-6_44

[101] Chen L et al. Expression of stromal cell-derived factor-1 in diabetic retinopathy. Chinese Medical Journal. 2010;**123**:984-988. DOI: 10.3760/cma.j.issn.0366-6999.2010.12.018

[102] Yu Y et al. The role of high mobility group box 1 (HMGB-1) in the diabetic retinopathy inflammation and apoptosis. International Journal of Clinical and Experimental Pathology. 2015;**8**:6807-6813. PMID: 26261566

[103] Victor A et al. Intercellular adhesive molecule-1 (ICAM-1) in proliferative diabetic retinopathy. 2016. (Unpublished data)

[104] Burgos R et al. Vitreous levels of IGF-I, IGF binding protein 1, and IGF binding protein 3 in proliferative diabetic retinopathy: A case-control study. Diabetes Care. 2000;**23**:80-83. DOI: 10.2337/diacare.24.3.516

[105] Tang S, Le-Ruppert KC, Gabel VP. Expression of intercellular adhesion molecule-1 (ICAM-1) and vascular cell adhesion molecule-1 (VCAM-1) on proliferating vascular endothelial cells in diabetic epiretinal membranes. The British Journal of Ophthalmology. 1994;**78**:370-376. PMID: 7517695

[106] Schröder S, Palinski W, Schmid-Schönbein GW. Activated monocytes and granulocytes, capillary nonperfusion, and neovascularization in diabetic retinopathy. The American Journal of Pathology. 1991;**139**:81-100. PMID: 1713023

[107] Patel N. Targeting leukostasis for the treatment of early diabetic retinopathy. Cardiovascular & Hematological Disorders Drug Targets. 2009;**9**:222-229. PMID: 19619127

[108] Hillier RJ et al. Aqueous humor cytokine levels as biomarkers of disease severity in diabetic macular edema. Retina. 2017;**37**:761-769. DOI: 10.1097/IAE.0000000000001210

[109] Yan Y et al. The impact of ranibizumab on the level of intercellular adhesion molecule type 1 in the vitreous of eyes with proliferative diabetic retinopathy. Acta Ophthalmologica. 2016;**94**:358-364. DOI: 10.1111/aos.12806

[110] Gustavsson C et al. Vascular cellular adhesion molecule-1 (VCAM-1) expression in mice retinal vessels is affected by both hyperglycemia and hyperlipidemia. PLoS One. 2010;**5**:e12699. DOI: 10.1371/journal.pone.0012699

[111] Lekaa A, Moemen MAA, Elhamid T, El Belltagi A. Contribution of vascular cell adhesion molecule 1 (VCAM-1) and erythropoietin (EPO) in the pathogenesis of proliferative diabetic retinopathy (PDR). Research Journal of Medicine and Medical Sciences. 2008;**3**:111-114

[112] Marui N et al. Vascular cell adhesion molecule-1 (VCAM-1) gene transcription and expression are regulated through an antioxidant-sensitive mechanism in human vascular endothelial cells. Journal of Clinical Investigation. 1993;**92**:1866-1874. DOI: 10.1172/JCI116778

[113] Semeraro F et al. Diabetic retinopathy: Vascular and inflammatory disease. Journal of Diabetes Research. 2015;**2015**:582060. DOI: 10.1155/2015/582060

[114] Adamiec-Mroczek J, Oficjalska-Młyńczak J, Misiuk-Hojło M. Proliferative diabetic retinopathy—The influence of diabetes control on the activation of the intraocular molecule system. Diabetes Research and Clinical Practice. 2009;**84**:46-50. DOI: 10.1016/j.diabres.2009.01.012

[115] Xu Y et al. Increased sCD200 levels in vitreous of patients with proliferative diabetic retinopathy and its correlation with vegf and proinflammatory cytokines. Investigative Opthalmology & Visual Science. 2015;**56**:6565. DOI: 10.1167/iovs.15-16854